Psychiatry

A Clinical Handbook

Mohsin Azam
Foundation Year One doctor, Royal Free Hospital, London

Mohammed Qureshi
Foundation Year Two doctor, Nottingham City Hospital

Daniel Kinnair
Consultant in General Adult Psychiatry, Leicester

Scion

© **Scion Publishing Ltd, 2016**

First published 2016

All rights reserved. No part of this book may be reproduced or transmitted, in any form or by any means, without permission.

A CIP catalogue record for this book is available from the British Library.

ISBN 978 1 907904 81 3

Scion Publishing Limited

The Old Hayloft, Vantage Business Park, Bloxham Road, Banbury OX16 9UX, UK

www.scionpublishing.com

Important Note from the Publisher

The information contained within this book was obtained by Scion Publishing Ltd from sources believed by us to be reliable. However, while every effort has been made to ensure its accuracy, no responsibility for loss or injury whatsoever occasioned to any person acting or refraining from action as a result of information contained herein can be accepted by the authors or publishers.

Readers are reminded that medicine is a constantly evolving science and while the authors and publishers have ensured that all dosages, applications and practices are based on current indications, there may be specific practices which differ between communities. You should always follow the guidelines laid down by the manufacturers of specific products and the relevant authorities in the country in which you are practising.

Although every effort has been made to ensure that all owners of copyright material have been acknowledged in this publication, we would be pleased to acknowledge in subsequent reprints or editions any omissions brought to our attention.

Registered names, trademarks, etc. used in this book, even when not marked as such, are not to be considered unprotected by law.

Line artwork by Hilary Strickland Illustration, Bath, UK

Typeset by Medlar Publishing Solutions Pvt Ltd, India

Printed in the UK

Contents

Preface

About a quarter of the population will experience some form of mental health issue in any given year, and as such, it is vitally important that medical students and junior doctors feel equipped to assess, diagnose and treat mental health conditions effectively. Whatever branch of medicine you end up practising, a thorough knowledge of mental health problems is becoming increasingly relevant.

There are a number of texts available to medical students and junior doctors; however, we set out to produce a book that provides comprehensive, up-to-date information, in a manner that is easily digestible. This book has been developed to support learners and equip them with the necessary knowledge of mental illnesses, their presentations, symptoms and appropriate management. Each chapter has been written to provide only the important key information about a particular psychiatric condition or concept, with invaluable reminders regarding what to look for in the history and mental state examination. Throughout the book, we have implemented a wide range of pedagogic features including figures, summary tables, illustrations and memory aids such as mnemonics. We also have dedicated chapters for single best answer questions and OSCE stations to aid revision for examinations.

There is no substitute for speaking to patients and developing your communication skills, but we anticipate that this book will strongly support you in enhancing these key skills. It is imperative that all doctors consider the impact of mental illness when seeing a patient, and the importance of a careful risk assessment. This clear and concise book will offer a greater insight into the absorbing branch of medicine that is psychiatry.

Mohsin Azam
Mohammed Qureshi
Daniel Kinnair
December 2015

Acknowledgements

We are very grateful to the medical students of the University of Leicester who gave invaluable suggestions with regard to the content and structure of the book.

We are also very grateful to Dr Karen Bretherton for her help in reviewing the chapter on autism and to Dr Girish Kunigiri for his assistance with the ECT chapter.

We would also like to place on record our sincere gratitude to the team at Scion Publishing Ltd for their great support, encouragement and patience.

Please refer to Appendix C for acknowledgements to the copyright holders of the images provided in this book.

Dedications

To my beloved grandmother, who recently left us having sadly suffered from Alzheimer's disease for many years. Your strength and determination have provided me with a great deal of inspiration and motivation.

My deepest appreciation goes to my parents. Without your continued support and encouragement, none of this would have been possible.

M.A.

To the two greatest inspirations in my life… Mum and Dad. No 'thank you' is great enough to repay you for all your support. I am so grateful to have you both in my life.

To my late grandparents whom I miss dearly.

And to Bashir… to the highest heavens my brother…

M.Q.

Abbreviations

6-CIT	6-item cognitive impairment test	COCP	combined oral contraceptive pill
β-hCG	beta human chorionic gonadotropin	COMT	catechol O-methyltransferase
AA	Alcoholics Anonymous	COPD	chronic obstructive pulmonary disease
ABCDE	airway, breathing, circulation, disability, exposure/examination	CPA	care programme approach
ABG	arterial blood gas	CPN	community psychiatric nurse
ABV	alcohol by volume	CRP	C-reactive protein
AC	approved clinician	CT	computed tomography
ACE	Addenbrooke's Cognitive Examination	CTO	community treatment order
		CVA	cerebrovascular accident
AD	Alzheimer's disease	CXR	chest X-ray
add+up	attention deficit disorders uniting parents	DBT	dialectical behavioural therapy
		DEXA	dual energy X-ray absorptiometry
ADDISS	Attention Deficit Disorder Information and Support Service	DLB	dementia with Lewy bodies
		DoLS	Deprivation of Liberty Safeguard
ADHD	attention deficit hyperactivity disorder	DSH	deliberate self-harm
		DSM	The APA classification of mental disorders
ADL	activities of daily living	DVLA	Driver & Vehicle Licensing Agency
A&E	Accident and Emergency	DVM	diurnal variation in mood
AKA	also known as	EAT	eating attitudes test
ALL	acute lymphocytic leukaemia	ECG	electocardiogram
AMHP	approved mental health professional	ECHO	echocardiogram
		ECT	electroconvulsive therapy
AML	acute myloid leukaemia	EDNOS	eating disorder not otherwise specified
AMT	Abbreviated Mental Test		
AN	anorexia nervosa	EEG	electroencephalogram
APA	American Psychiatric Asssociation	EMDR	eye movement desensitization and reprocessing
ASD	autism spectrum disorders		
AUDIT	Alcohol Use Disorders Identification Test	EPSE	extrapyramidal side effects
		ERP	exposure and response prevention
AVPU	alert, voice, pain, unresponsive	FBC	full blood count
AXR	abdominal X-ray	FSH	follicle-stimulating hormone
BD	twice daily (*bis die*)	GABA	gamma-aminobutyric acid
BDNF	brain-derived neurotrophic factor	GAD	generalized anxiety disorder
		GCS	Glasgow coma scale
BN	bulimia nervosa	GHB	gamma-hydroxybutyrate
BNF	*British National Formulary*	GI	gastrointestinal
BP	blood pressure	GP	general practitioner
BPAD	bipolar affective disorder	GPCOG	General Practitioner Assessment of Cognition
BZD	benzodiazepines		
CAM	Confusion Assessment Method	HbA1c	glycated haemoglobin
CAT	cognitive analytic therapy	HPA	hypothalamic–pituitary–adrenal
CBT	cognitive behavioural therapy	HR	heart rate
CCF	congestive cardiac failure	IAPT	improving access to psychological therapies
CJD	Creutzfeldt–Jakob disease		
CMHT	community mental health team	ICD	International Classification of Diseases
CMV	cytomegalovirus		
CNS	central nervous system	ICE	ideas, concerns and expectations

Abbreviations

ICP	intra-cranial pressure
IMCA	independent mental capacity advocate
IN	intranasal
IPT	interpersonal therapy
IQ	intelligence quotient
IV	intravenous
LD	learning disability
LFTs	liver function tests
LH	luteinizing hormone
MAO	monoamine oxidase
MAOI	monoamine oxidase inhibitor
MCA	Mental Capacity Act
MCV	mean cell volume
MDMA	methylenedioxymethamphetamine
MDT	multidisciplinary team
MHA	Mental Health Act
MHAC	Mental Health Act Commission
MI	myocardial infarction
MMPI	Minnesota Multiphasic Personality Inventory
MMR	measles, mumps, rubella
MMSE	Mini-Mental State Examination
MOCA	Montreal Cognitive Assessment
MRI	magnetic resonance imaging
MSE	mental state examination
MSU	midstream specimen of urine
N+V	nausea and vomiting
NARI	noradrenaline reuptake inhibitor
NAS	National Autistic Society
NASSA	noradrenaline-serotonin specific antidepressant
NMDA	N-methyl-D-aspartate
NICE	National Institute for Health and Care Excellence
NKDA	no known drug allergies
NPIS	National Poisons Information Service
NR	nearest relative
OCD	obsessive–compulsive disorder
OD	once daily (omni die)
OGD	oesophago-gastro duodenoscopy
OSCE	objective structured clinical examinations
OT	occupational therapist
OTC	over the counter

PANDAS	paediatric autoimmune neuro-psychiatric disorders associated with streptococcal infections
PD	personality disorder
PE	psychoeducation
PKU	phenylketonuria
PO	oral (per os)
PRN	when required (pro re nata)
PT	prothrombin time
PTSD	post-traumatic stress disorder
QDS	four times a day (quater die sumendum)
RC	responsible clinician
RR	respiratory rate
SADQ	Severity of Alcohol Dependence Questionnaire
SARI	serotonin antagonist and reuptake inhibitor
SBA	single best answer
SNRI	serotonin and noradrenaline reuptake inhibitor
SNS	sympathetic nervous system
SOAD	second opinion appointed doctor
SPECT	single-photon emission computerized tomography
SSRI	selective serotonin reuptake inhibitor
TASR	Tool for Assessment of Suicide Risk
TB	tuberculosis
TCA	tricyclic antidepressant
TFTs	thyroid function tests
ToF	tetralogy of Fallot
ToRCH	toxoplasmosis, other (syphilis, varicella-zoster, parvovirus B19), rubella, cytomegalovirus (CMV), and herpes
TSQ	trauma screening questionnaire
U&Es	urea and electrolytes
UTI	urinary tract infection
VaD	vascular dementia
VBG	venous blood gas
VDRL	venereal disease research laboratory (test for syphilis)
VSD	ventricular septal defect
WCC	white cell count
WHO	World Health Organization
Y-BOCS	Yale–Brown obsessive–compulsive scale

Outline of the book

- Explains the concept of psychiatry, its relevance in modern-day healthcare and reasons behind studying it. Highlights the book's usefulness for medical students, junior doctors, psychiatric trainees, GP trainees and psychiatric nurses.
- Delves briefly into the history of psychiatry as well as key concepts including psychiatric classification systems, the community mental health team (multidisciplinary team) and the bio-psychosocial approach. Furthermore, a mind map illustrates all of the psychiatric disorders covered in this book, which are principally based on the ICD-10 criteria.

Chapter 2: Assessment in psychiatry

- Discusses in depth the two key components of the psychiatric assessment: the psychiatric history and the mental state examination.
- These chapters are packed with hints and tips that can be applied clinically and in OSCEs.

Chapters 3–11: The psychiatric disorders

- A detailed overview of all the psychiatric conditions. A bullet point format is used, with key information in bold, making the valuable points easy to identify.
- For each condition, the following areas will be discussed:
  - Definition: A concise definition will be stated for each condition with key words in **bold** to emphasize their importance.
  - Pathophysiology/Aetiology: Pathophysiology and aetiology often overlap and as such we have placed them together in the same section. All psychiatric conditions are multifactorial in their development, and we aim to divide this section into categories for ease of recall, most commonly biological and environmental.
  - Epidemiology and risk factors: Up to date sources have been used to highlight the incidence and prevalence of the psychiatric disorders. Risk factors are also listed, where relevant, in order of importance.
  - Clinical features: Clinical features are described for all conditions, with helpful use of images, figures and mnemonics where appropriate.
  - Diagnosis and investigations: This section covers four valuable sub-sections. Firstly, an area dedicated to history taking includes specific questions articulated to assist you in a clinical situation (often a psychiatric line of questioning is sensitive in nature, with questions needing to be phrased cautiously). Secondly, we delve into the mental state examination (MSE) findings specific to the condition in question. Thirdly, we cite the investigations required to help with diagnosis, with justification offered for all. Finally, we cover the differential diagnoses for the condition (*see below* for associated symbols used in the book).

History taking	Mental state examination	Investigations	Differential diagnosis
Hx	MSE	Ix	DDx

- **Management:** The final section explores the management of the respective conditions. We deploy the use of the bio-psychosocial model in order to divide management strategies into specific strata. NICE (National Institute for Health and Care Excellence) guidelines have been used to provide the most reliable and comprehensive information. The *BNF* (*British National Formulary*) has been used where pharmacological aspects of management have been discussed.
- At the end of each chapter 'self-assessment questions' are provided in the form of short answer questions. These questions are specifically designed to see whether readers have grasped the information provided for each condition and are also an opportunity for students to practise answering exam-style short answer questions.
- Special features include:

OSCE tips	OSCE tip boxes offer helpful hints and tips that will enable you to perform well in OSCE settings.
Key facts	Key fact boxes discuss important points that you are more likely to be tested on in your exams.
ICD-10 Criteria	The clinical features section has an ICD-10 criteria box to list the clinical features and relevant timing of these features required for diagnosing a psychiatric condition.
'MNEMONIC'	We provide invaluable mnemonics throughout the textbook, for various areas we feel that students struggle to recall but are absolutely crucial to know.

Chapter 12: Management

Including key information on:

- **Psychotherapy:** key information including indications, rationale, aim and modes of delivery is provided for the most commonly used psychotherapies, including cognitive behavioural therapy and psychodynamic therapy. Many other forms of simpler and relatively new psychotherapy are also discussed.
- **Pharmacology:** key information (including examples, indications, mechanisms of action, side effects, contraindications and route and dose) on antidepressants, mood stabilizers, antipsychotics, hypnotics and anxiolytics is provided. We use **DO** and **DO NOT** boxes to highlight important points to bear in mind when initiating pharmacological agents in psychiatry.
- **Electroconvulsive therapy (ECT):** the following key information is provided for ECT therapy: definition, background information including a brief history, what ECT involves, indications, side effects and contraindications.
- **Mental health and the law:** A review of mental health and the law in England and Wales, including the Mental Health Act and the Mental Capacity Act, is provided. The most salient points are highlighted as this topic commonly crops up in examinations.

Chapter 13: Forensic psychiatry

- This brief chapter discusses the assessment and treatment of offenders with mental health disorders. We also mention the considerations during court proceedings and predictors of violent behaviour.

Chapter 14: Common OSCE scenarios and mark schemes

- Being as student friendly as possible we delve into five common OSCE scenarios, likely to appear in exams.
- These should ideally be practised in a group of three, with a student, simulated patient and assessor.
- We also provide a detailed mark scheme check list.

Chapter 15: Exam-style questions

- A selection of 40 single best answer (SBA) questions are provided that will challenge your knowledge. SBAs have been specifically chosen – they are the style of questions most commonly used across medical schools in the UK.

Glossary of terms

- Definitions of the key terms and concepts mentioned throughout the course of the book are provided in the glossary. Key words can be looked up swiftly without having to spend time sieving them out!

Appendices

- Answers to the exam-style questions are given with detailed explanation and justification of the method for reaching the correct answer.
- Detailed answers are also provided for the self-assessment questions at the end of the section for each psychiatric condition.

Chapter 1

Introduction to psychiatry

What is psychiatry?

- Psychiatry is the branch of medicine that deals with the diagnosis, treatment and prevention of mental, emotional and behavioural disorders.
- It is one of the most varied specialties in medicine. Psychiatrists can work in a number of settings including the hospital, nursing homes, community settings, people's own homes and even prisons.
- Different areas of psychiatry include: general adult psychiatry; child and adolescent psychiatry; psychiatry of old age; learning disability psychiatry; forensic psychiatry; addiction psychiatry; social and rehabilitation psychiatry; psychotherapy; eating disorder psychiatry; and liaison psychiatry.
- Mental illness is very common. Research suggests that **1 in 4** people will experience a mental health problem over the course of a year. The prevalence of this set of conditions ranks alongside cardiovascular diseases and malignancies.

History of psychiatry

- The history of psychiatry dates back to as early as the Ancient Egyptian Empire. However, it is only since the turn of the twentieth century that psychiatry as we know it today, has begun to take shape. See *Fig. 1.1* for notable events in psychiatry.
- The late 1940s, with the discovery of lithium to stabilize moods, and the early 1950s, with chlorpromazine as the first antipsychotic, ushered in the new era of psychopharmacology.

Why study psychiatry?

- Psychiatry is an enthralling and dynamic specialty. Studying psychiatry is important for medical students as it is a frequent exam topic both in written papers and the practical assessment.
- Moreover, psychiatric issues, for instance depression, anxiety and personality disorders, are prominent in many areas of medicine, but often overlooked. Therefore it is imperative for all healthcare professionals to have knowledge of the impact of mental health disorders.
- General practice and A&E are areas of medicine where psychiatric conditions are common. In primary care, roughly **20–25%** of patients seen suffer from a psychiatric disorder, either in isolation or accompanying physical illness.
- Psychiatric illness can also affect physical health. There is a **10–25 year reduction in life expectancy** (premature mortality) for patients with severe psychiatric disorders (*WHO*) (*Fig. 1.2*). The vast majority of these deaths are due to chronic physical health conditions such as cardiovascular, respiratory and infectious diseases, diabetes and hypertension. Suicide is another important cause of death. Health risk behaviours such as smoking are more common.
- The content in this textbook will provide useful information not only for medical students, but for junior doctors, GP trainees and psychiatric nurses. The information in this book will provide you with:
  - A basic understanding of the common psychiatric disorders encountered not only by psychiatrists, but rather in a variety of healthcare settings.
  - Knowledge of how to perform a comprehensive and efficient psychiatric assessment including the psychiatric history and mental state examination.
  - Information on how to manage a patient holistically by adopting the mantra of the bio-psychosocial approach, which is a transferable skill amongst all specialties.

1550BC: The Ebers Papyrus, one of the most important medical manuscripts of Ancient Egypt, describes disorders such as depression and dementia.

400BC: Ancient Greek physician Hippocrates hypothesizes that physiological abnormalities cause mental problems.

705AD: First psychiatric hospital built by Muslims in Baghdad.

1247: Europe's first mental health institution, Bethlem Royal Hospital (then referred to as Bedlam asylum), is established. Unstable patients were commonly chained up.

1808: The word 'psychiatry' was first used by Johann Christian Reil in a 188-page paper.

1845: The Lunacy Act passed in England enhancing status of mentally ill persons to patients.

1893: German psychiatrist Emil Kraepelin clinically defines what would later become known as schizophrenia.

1901: Alois Alzheimer identifies the first case of what became known as Alzheimer's disease.

1917: Sigmund Freud publishes one of his most famous works, *Introduction to Psychoanalysis*, outlining his theory of neuroses.

1948: Lithium bicarbonate's ability to stabilize mood swings cited by Australian psychiatrist John Cade.

1951: First antipsychotic, chlorpromazine, is developed.

1960: Aaron Beck develops cognitive therapy.

1977: ICD-9 published by the World Health Organization.

1988: Fluoxetine, the first SSRI, is released for treatment of depression.

Fig. 1.1: Notable events in the history of psychiatry.

Psychiatric classification

- The **International Classification of Diseases (ICD)** is the standard diagnostic tool for epidemiology, health management and clinical purposes (***World Health Organization***).

- The two main classification systems for mental disorders are the **ICD-10** and **DSM-V** (produced by the American Psychiatric Association).

NOTE: For the purposes of this textbook, we will be strictly using ICD-10 criteria as this system predominates in the UK.

- ICD-10 divides mental and behavioural disorders into **ten categories**: (1) F00–F09 **Organic, including symptomatic, mental disorders**; (2) F10–F19 **Mental and behavioural disorders** due to use of **psychoactive substances**; (3) F20–F29 **Schizophrenia, schizotypal and delusional disorders**; (4) F30–F39 **Mood [affective] disorders**; (5) F40–F48 **Neurotic, stress-related and somatoform disorders**; (6) F50–F59 **Behavioural syndromes** associated with physiological disturbances and physical factors; (7) F60–F69 **Disorders of personality and behaviour in adult persons**; (8) F70–F79 **Mental retardation**; (9) F80–F89 Disorders of **psychological development**; (10) F90–F98 **Behavioural and emotional disorders** with onset usually occurring in **childhood and adolescence**.

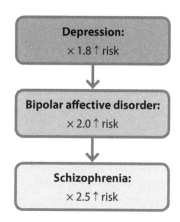

Fig. 1.2: ↑ risk of mortality in the major psychiatric disorders vs. the general population.

Areas of psychiatry

Psychiatry is a broad specialty with many distinct and varying conditions (*Fig. 1.3*).

Psychiatric assessment

Formulating a psychiatric diagnosis is a structured process involving an initial assessment, generating differential diagnoses, and then performing investigations to come to a diagnosis.

Initial assessment

- **Psychiatric history:** see *Section 2.1*.
- **Mental state examination:** see *Section 2.2*.
- **Physical examination:** Certain medical conditions (e.g. anaemia, thyroid abnormalities) can present with psychiatric features. If alcohol abuse is suspected, the physical signs which accompany it must be assessed for.

Differential diagnosis

- **Organic:** Due to demonstrable pathology of the brain, e.g. delirium, dementia and substance related disorders.
- **Functional:** Any non-organic condition. Have predominantly psychological causes, e.g. psychoses such as schizophrenia or mood disorders such as depression.
- **Personality disorders**.

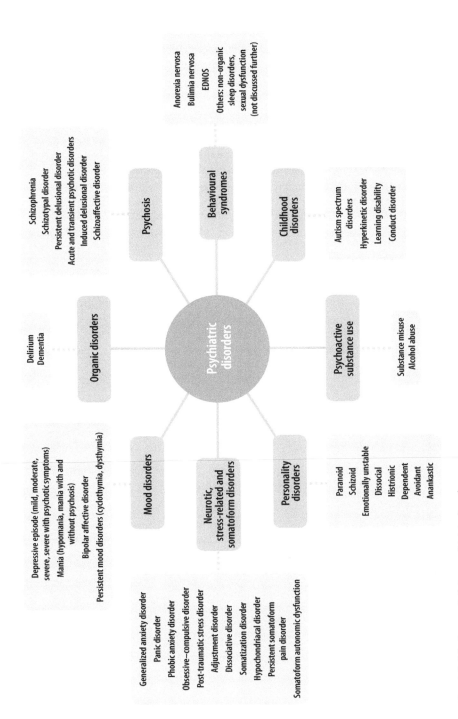

Fig. 1.3: Mind map of all the psychiatric disorders.

Investigations

- **Biochemical testing:** Include blood tests or urine tests (e.g. for substance misuse).
- **Imaging:** Such as CT head (in dementia) or chest radiograph (in delirium where underlying pneumonia is suspected).
- **Questionnaires:** Various questionnaires exist for conditions such as depressive disorders, anxiety disorders and dementia.

The multidisciplinary team (MDT)

- In the UK, psychiatric care is becoming more **community based** with patients being treated in outpatient clinics, day hospitals or their own homes where possible (*Fig. 1.4*).
- A key concept is that of the **Community Mental Health Team (CMHT)** which is a **multidisciplinary team** designed to manage patients with psychiatric conditions in the community, and ultimately to prevent emergency admission to hospital. There is a designated **care coordinator** (or key worker) and a **care plan** records identified needs. Both General Adult Psychiatry and Older Persons Psychiatry services may have CMHTs as part of their community mental health provision (see *Table 1.1*).

Table 1.1: The roles of different mental health professionals in the CMHT	
Psychiatrist	The consultant is the clinical leader of the team and responsible for psychiatric assessment and management. Initiates and supervises pharmacological treatment and may provide psychological intervention. There are also registrars who contribute to outpatient clinics and junior doctors who assist in management of inpatients.
Community psychiatric nurse (CPN)	A central member of the team who reviews patients in their residences, or in clinic settings. Usually key workers for patients with chronic mental disorders. May provide counselling and monitor efficacy of treatments and side effects. May administer depot injections but cannot prescribe medications.
Occupational therapist	Offers functional assessment of independence in ADL, and provides skills training. May assist patient in finding an occupation.
Social worker	Performs social assessments and assists patients in meeting their housing and financial needs. Looks for suitable placements (residential or nursing care depending on nursing needs, e.g. continence, mobility), for example in dementia patients.
Clinical psychologist	Carries out psychological assessment and the full range of psychological treatments.
Secretary/ Administrator	Arranges outpatient appointments. Organizes and coordinates weekly CMHT meetings.

Crisis resolution team

- Set up to manage severely unwell and often suicidal psychiatric patients in the community.
- Essentially deal with psychiatric emergencies. The service is available 24 hours a day and visits can occur daily.
- The focus of this team is short-term interventions (usually not more than 6 weeks) with people at home, to prevent admission to hospital.

Outreach team

- Provide intensive support and treatment in the community for chronically unwell psychiatric patients and those who have a history of disengagement from mainstream psychiatric services.
- The patients are usually at high risk of causing harm to themselves or others.
- Community nurses can visit several times a week over a long period of time.

Community mental health team (CMHT) (see *Table 1.1*)

- This is a multidisciplinary team formed between psychiatrists, community psychiatric nurses (CPN), occupational therapists, psychologists, social workers and secretaries.
- These constituent members work as a seamless unit in order to ensure optimal care for patients from a psychiatric and social point of view.
- CPNs may visit people at home once a fortnight, and patients can also be seen in outpatient clinic settings.

Care programme approach (CPA)

- A system of care which aims to meet a patient's psychiatric and social needs once they are back in the community after significant contact with psychiatric services (e.g. an inpatient admission).
- Medical and social services work together closely and a member of the CMHT is appointed as a care coordinator (or key worker).
- Patients open to psychiatric services may be under the CPA if they have complex needs, or where multiple services need coordinating.

Early intervention in psychosis team

- Work with young people (usually under the age of 35) in their first episode of psychosis.
- Provide interventions targeted at ↓ the duration of untreated psychosis (a strong prognostic indicator).

Fig. 1.4: Key psychiatric concepts in the community.

Bio-psychosocial approach

- The **bio-psychosocial model**, theorized by the psychiatrist George Engel, is the mainstream ideology of contemporary psychiatry.
- According to the model, health is best understood as a combination of biological, psychological and social factors as opposed to earlier, purely biological ideas.
- Throughout this book we will utilize the bio-psychosocial approach, particularly in the context of management of psychiatric illness (*Fig. 1.5*).

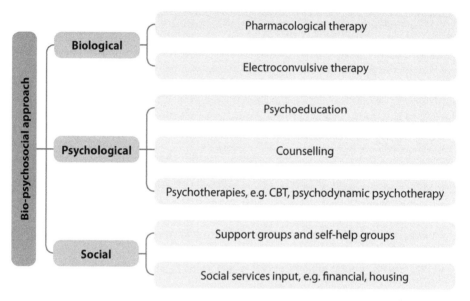

Fig. 1.5: Bio-psychosocial approach to management in psychiatry.

Chapter 2

Assessment in psychiatry

Introduction to psychiatric history taking

- Taking a psychiatric history is structurally similar to a medical history. The major differences are in the **social** and **developmental history** (also known as the **personal history**), which are covered in more depth, as well as the **past psychiatric history**.
- A thorough psychiatric history takes approximately **1 hour**. You may find it helpful to jot down notes as you go along, as this can aid you in being more methodical in your history taking.
- The areas you need to cover in the history are shown in *Fig. 2.1.1*.
- It is not always appropriate to ask all of the questions in every single case presentation. It can sometimes be more prudent to leave gaps to fill in later, particularly if your patient is suspicious, paranoid, or acutely distressed.
- Parts of the history can be found in the old notes, as well as a **collateral history** from an informant.
- As with any history, it is important to begin with open-ended questions and focus in on certain areas with more specific, closed questions. This gives the patient a chance to talk about their experiences and concerns, whilst allowing you to gain the information you need.
- As with any medical history, at the conclusion you should be able to generate a list of differential diagnoses based on the symptoms you have elicited during the history taking.
- Everyone has their own style of interviewing and there is no single 'correct way'. However, you need to feel comfortable with the style you adopt, so that the sensitive questions are not phrased awkwardly.

Before the interview (the 4 S's)

- **Site:** Ideally the room should be as **comfortable** and sound proof as can be, but this is not always possible on wards or in the emergency department.
- **Safety:** It is important that you sit closer to the door than your patients and in some cases, a chaperone may be required. Check local added precautions such as panic buttons and alarms.
- **Setting:** It is best to arrange chairs at 90° to each other. If a desk is required to make notes, this should not be directly in between the patient and the interviewer such that it is obstructing. Sit in a relaxed posture. Ensure that there are no interruptions by turning mobile phones off and handing bleeps to colleagues.
- **Study:** Read any referral letter or previous notes to familiarize yourself with the case. Take any appropriate collateral history from a member of staff or family.

Psychiatric history
↓
Introduce yourself
↓
Identifying information
↓
Reason for referral
↓
Presenting complaint
↓
Ideas, Concerns and Expectations
↓
Past psychiatric history
↓
Past medical history
↓
Drug history
↓
Family history
↓
Personal history
↓
Social history
↓
Premorbid personality

Fig. 2.1.1: Components of the psychiatric history.

Introduction

- Introduce yourself including your **name** and your **role**.
- Explain the **purpose** of the consultation and how long you have to interview the patient.
- Gain **consent** to take a history and ask for permission to take notes.

Identifying information ('NAG MORE')

- **N**ame (full)
- **A**ge
- **G**ender
- **M**arital status and children
- **O**ccupation (present and past)
- **R**eligious and **E**thnic background

NOTE: Some of this information may be gathered during the history, or from the medical notes. We would avoid covering all of this in a conversation with the patient before asking about the presenting complaint.

Reason for referral

- **WHEN** was the patient admitted (date and time)?
- **WHY** was the patient admitted?
- **WHO** was involved in the patient's admission, e.g. GP, A&E, police, social worker?
- Is the patient in hospital voluntarily or detained under the Mental Health Act?

Presenting complaint

- Start with an **open-ended question**, for example 'How can we help you?' or 'How have you been feeling?'
- Onset: 'When did you realize things have changed?'
- Severity: 'How has this affected your life?'
- Duration: 'How long has this been going on for?'
- Progression: 'Have you had any fluctuations in the way you have been feeling?'
- Precipitating events/Aggravating and relieving factors: 'Has anything occurred in your life recently which could explain how you are feeling?'
- Associated symptoms: Always screen for depression, psychosis and suicidal ideation.

OSCE tips 1: Controlling the consultation

If the patient has:
- **Anxiety** → Reassure and normalize their symptoms.
- **Mania** → Try focusing them on the purpose of the interview, explain that you are interrupting to re-direct them and will come back to what they are saying later.
- **Confusion** (delirium or dementia) → Try to orientate the patient to time and place.
- **Psychosis** → Be empathetic and non-judgemental and acknowledge non-verbal cues (e.g. responses to hallucinations).

OSCE tips 2: Screening for other psychiatric disorders (*Table 2.1.1*)

In any psychiatric history, it is important to screen for the main psychiatric problems (e.g. depression and psychosis) even if the patient comes in with a different presenting complaint. Keep it as brief as possible, asking about the main symptoms, e.g. for depression ask about the core symptoms and for psychosis ask about the presence of delusions and hallucinations.

Table 2.1.1: Specific presenting complaints and how to phrase questions accordingly	
Depression	
Low mood	'Have you noticed any changes in your mood recently?'
Anhedonia	'Do you still enjoy the things that you used to enjoy?', 'Is there anything that you enjoy or that makes you happy?'
Anergia	'How would you describe your energy levels?', 'On a scale of 1 to 10 with 1 being extremely tired and 10 being full of energy, where would you place yourself?'
Psychosis	
Delusions	'Do you have any specific worries at the moment?', 'Do you feel safe or are you in any danger?' (**persecutory delusion**)
Hallucinations	Make sure you signpost: 'I want to ask you about experiences which people sometimes have, but find difficult to talk about. These are questions I ask everyone.', 'Do you ever see (**visual**) or hear (**auditory**) things that other people seem unable to see or hear?'
Auditory hallucinations	'Are the voices/people talking about you (**third person**) or directly to you (**second person**), are they commenting on what you are doing (third person – **running commentary**) or are they telling you to do certain things? If so, what are they telling you?'
Anxiety	
Generalized anxiety	'Would you say you were an anxious person?', 'Do you feel particularly anxious or on edge?', 'Do you worry about day to day things?', 'Do you feel irritable often?', 'Do you find that you are unable to relax?'
Panic attacks	'Do you ever suffer from shortness of breath/chest pain/palpitations/ sweating/ tremor?', 'How long do attacks last?', 'Is there anything which triggers these episodes?'
Phobias	'Do you have any fears that you or others may consider to be irrational?', 'Do you have any thoughts that you would consider obsessive?'
Obsessions	'Do any thoughts or worries keep coming back to your mind even though you try to push them away?'

Ideas, concerns and expectations (ICE)

ICE is a crucial part of the history. Eliciting health beliefs and concerns in a sincere and fluent manner will enable you to build a strong rapport with the patient.

- **Ideas:** 'Do you have any thoughts as to what could be making you feel this way?'
- **Concerns:** 'Is there anything that is particularly concerning or worrying you at the moment?'
- **Expectations:** 'Do you have any thoughts as to the best way in which you feel we can help you?'

OSCE tips 3: Watch out for non-verbal cues!

Picking up on **non-verbal cues** is essential when taking a psychiatric history. Although the mental state examination is specifically targeted towards this, your examination essentially starts as soon as you see the patient. For instance, patients with depression often have poor eye contact whereas patients with psychosis may respond to auditory or visual hallucinations and it is very important to register this.

Past psychiatric history

- Have there been any similar problems to the presenting complaint, in the past? Previous or ongoing **psychiatric diagnoses** – 'Do you have any psychiatric illness that you are aware of?'
- **Dates** and **duration** of previous episodes of mental illness.
- Whether or not the **Mental Health Act** was ever implemented.
- Details of previous **hospitalization** and **treatment** including medications, psychotherapy and electroconvulsive therapy. Ask about **response to treatment** and about **side effects**.

Past medical history and drug history

- Ask about any current or previous **medical illnesses** or any past **surgical procedures:** 'Is there anything that you are currently seeing the doctor for?'
- Ask particularly about **head injuries** and **previous cranial surgery**, **neurological conditions** (e.g. epilepsy) and **endocrine abnormalities** (e.g. thyroid disease).
- Find out about **medication** the patient is using (both prescription and over-the-counter). Also, ask specifically about previous use of **psychotropic medication**, and whether the reported medication helped symptoms or caused side effects.
- Enquire about **allergies**, including the **nature** of any allergy (e.g. rash, anaphylaxis).

OSCE tips 4: Be careful not to offend patients

A psychiatric history contains extremely sensitive questions and it is important not to cause offence to the patient as this can make the consultation counterproductive. There are tools designed to aid you with this:
1. **Signposting** → 'I'm sorry to have to ask you this…' or 'It is important to ask you the following which we ask everyone…'
2. **Normalizing** → 'Some people can feel this way…has this happened to you?'
3. **Acknowledge embarrassment** → 'I know this is a sensitive topic…'

This will help establish and build a good rapport with the patient.

Family history

- Presence of **psychiatric illness in family members:** 'Has anyone in your family ever suffered from problems like you're having now?'
- **Quality of family relationships:** Collect information about parents, siblings and other significant relatives. 'How do you get on with your family?', 'Are there any recent significant events that have occurred in the family?'
- Brief **medical history of family:** 'Are there any medical conditions which run in the family?'
- It can be very useful to draw a **genogram** to represent information appropriately.

Personal history (*Table 2.1.2*)

- The **personal history** is crucial in identifying **predisposing factors** to the patient's psychiatric illnesses (*Fig. 2.1.2*).

Table 2.1.2: Personal history	
Early childhood	• **Antenatal and intrapartum complications:** 'When your mother had you, are you aware of any complications during the pregnancy or at birth?' • **Developmental milestones:** 'As far as you are aware, did you walk and talk at the right ages, or were you a slow developer?' • **Childhood illness:** 'Were you frequently unwell as a child, or often in hospital as a baby?' • **Childhood psychiatric illness:** 'As a young child do you feel that you were unusually aggressive or struggled with social interaction?' • **Family dynamics:** 'Were your parents married when they had you?', 'Were you planned?', 'Do you have any siblings or step-siblings?' • **Home atmosphere:** 'What is your earliest memory?', 'Was it a happy one?' • **Childhood abuse:** 'Have you ever had any unpleasant experiences in childhood, such as sexual, psychological or physical abuse?'
Education	• 'Did you attend mainstream or specialist schools?' • 'Did you enjoy school? If not, why?' • 'Were you ever bullied at school?' • 'Were you ever told that you had behavioural problems during school?' • 'Did you finish school?' • 'Did you attend higher education and what qualifications have you achieved?'
Employment	• **Chronological list of jobs:** 'Where have worked so far (in order)?' • **Duration of work:** 'How long did you work for in each job?' • **Redundancy or personal choice:** 'Why did you move on from a particular job?' • **Work environment:** 'How would you describe your relationship with your boss and co-workers?'
Relationships	• **Sexual orientation:** 'How would you describe your sexuality? Are you heterosexual, homosexual or bisexual?' • **Chronological account of major relationships:** 'Would you be able to give me an account of the major relationships you've had in your life?' • **Current relationship:** 'Are you currently in a relationship?' • **Children:** 'Do you have any children from current or previous relationships?', 'Who do the children live with?', 'Could you describe your relationship with your children?'
Forensic history	• 'Have you ever been charged with, or convicted of, any offences?' • If the answer to the above is yes, 'What sentence did you receive?' • 'Do you have any outstanding charges or convictions at present?'

NOTE: In the case of **women** the interviewer should ask about menstrual patterns and previous miscarriages, stillbirths or terminations.

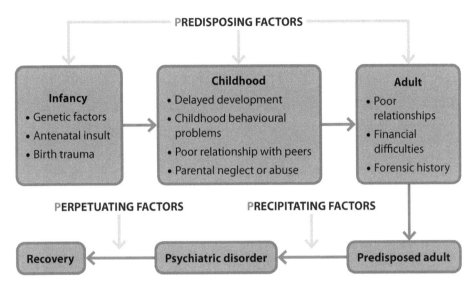

Fig. 2.1.2: Aetiological factors in psychiatric illness can be divided into the three Ps (Predisposing, Precipitating and Perpetuating factors). The predisposing factors highlight the importance of taking a personal history.

Social history

- This includes current **accommodation** (state of housing, heating, living conditions), **social support** (friends and family), **financial circumstances** (any debts or benefits) and **hobbies** or **leisure activities**.

Alcohol and substance misuse

- The **CAGE questionnaire** is a useful tool to screen for **alcohol dependence** → if two or more positive, see if they meet alcohol dependence syndrome (see *Section 7.2*, Alcohol abuse).
- How much **alcohol** in a day (units consumed) and type of alcohol.
- Use of **illicit drugs:** 'Have you ever used any recreational drugs?'
- Record **drug names**, **routes** of administration and **years/frequency** of use: 'How much do you spend on this in a week?'
- **Smoking** status: Calculate the **pack-year** smoking history
  (Number of cigarettes smoked per day × duration of smoking in years) ÷ 20

NOTE: The 20 in this equation is the number of cigarettes in a pack.

Premorbid personality

- The **premorbid personality** is an assessment of the patient's personality and character *before* the onset of mental illness.
- 'How would people have described you before?', 'Would they describe you differently now?'
- It may be useful to gain a **collateral history** from a family member or friend about premorbid personality in order to corroborate the patient's account.

Summary

- Succinctly **summarize** your understanding of what the patient has told you.
- Provide an opportunity for the patient to ask **questions**.

OSCE tips 5: Psychiatric history summarized

1. **Introductory information:** Age, sex, occupation, ethnic background, marital status.
2. **Reason for referral:** When was the patient admitted, why was the patient admitted and by whom?
3. **Presenting complaint** and **history of presenting complaint:** Onset, severity, duration, precipitating events, associated symptoms.
4. **Past psychiatric history:** Nature, date and duration of previous mental disorders, names of doctors and hospitals, outcomes, history of self-harm, attempted suicide and risk to others.
5. **Past medical history** and **drug history:** Co-morbid physical illness, past and childhood illnesses, surgery, medications (dose, route, side effects) including over-the-counter. Allergies, including type of reaction.
6. **Family history:** Anyone in family suffering from or previously suffered from a mental disorder, alcohol or drug dependency, self-harm or attempted suicide?
7. **Social history:** Self-care, family and social support, finances, smoking, alcohol, illicit drugs.
8. **Personal history:** Early childhood, education, employment, relationships, forensic history.
9. **Premorbid personality:** Personality and character *before* the onset of mental illness.

OSCE tips 6: An example of presenting your psychiatric history

This is Mr X, a 35-year-old man who presents with a 3-month history of low mood, anhedonia and lack of energy, along with biological symptoms of weight loss, reduced libido and early morning wakening. There are no psychotic features and there is no current suicidal ideation. He has no previous psychiatric history and no past history of self-harm or suicidal acts, and is otherwise medically fit on no regular medication and with no significant family history. There is no history of significant alcohol or substance misuse. In conclusion, Mr X is likely to be suffering from a severe depressive disorder and I would like to commence with my mental state examination to further explore Mr X's current mental state, to explore his risk further and to further support my conclusions from the history.

2.2 Mental state examination

Introduction

- The mental state examination (MSE) is a systematic appraisal of the appearance, behaviour, mental functioning and overall demeanour of a person. In other words, it reflects a person's psychological functioning at a given point in time.
- The MSE is usually put into a time frame (e.g. the preceding 2 weeks).
- The history and mental state examination will lead to the formation of differential diagnoses.
- Most of us inherently perform many aspects of the MSE every time we interact with, or observe others.
- Observations of the mental state are important in determining a person's capacity to function, and whether psychiatric follow-up is required.
- Judgements about mental state should always consider the developmental level of the patient and age-appropriateness of the noted behaviour.
- If there is any indication of current suicidal or homicidal ideation, then the person must be urgently referred for assessment by a qualified mental health clinician.
- An MSE includes the following eight areas: **appearance**, **behaviour**, **speech**, **mood**, **thought**, **perception**, **cognition** and **insight**.

> **OSCE tips 1:** A useful mnemonic for the MSE: '**ASEPTIC**'
>
> **A**ppearance and behaviour
> **S**peech
> **E**motion (mood)
> **P**erception
> **T**houghts
> **I**nsight
> **C**ognition

Appearance and behaviour

- **Physical state:** What age does the patient appear? Ethnic origin? Do they appear physically unwell? Are they sweating? Are they unkempt? What is their weight? Any extrapyramidal side effects from antipsychotics? Posture (hunched in depression or upright in anxiety)?
- **Clothing and accessories:** Flamboyant, bright clothing in mania. Dirty, stained or torn clothing in depression, schizophrenia, substance misuse and dementia.
- **Personal hygiene:** Self-neglect in substance misuse, depression, schizophrenia.
- **Eye contact:** Inappropriate eye contact (staring in parkinsonism), averting gaze (depression).
- **Facial expression:** Tearful (depression), overly happy (mania).
- **Body language:** Relaxed, tense or withdrawn. Comment on how the body language might have changed during the consultation.
- **Motor activity and abnormal movements:** Psychomotor retardation (slowing of movements) in depression. Agitation may be seen in manic states, or when distressed. Examples of abnormal movements include tardive dyskinesia and acute dystonia (typical antipsychotics), tremor (anxiety disorders or lithium toxicity), catatonia (schizophrenia), tics (Tourette's syndrome).
- **Level of arousal:** Calm or agitated (delirium, mania).
- **Ability to build rapport:** Can be affected by factors relating to the patient and by how the interviewer manages the conversation.
- **Disinhibition:** e.g. in fronto-temporal dementia, hypomania, mania.

Speech

- **Rate:** Rapid and pressured (mania), mumbling and slow (depression, dementia).
- **Rhythm:** Normal, flattened or ↑ intonation (the pattern of pitch changes in connected speech).
- **Volume:** Loud (mania), normal, quiet (depression).
- **Content:** Excessive punning (mania), clang association (ideas that are related only by similar or rhyming sounds rather than actual meaning), monosyllabic (a vocabulary composed primarily of monosyllables), spontaneous speech or only in answer to questions.
- **Quantity:** Increased (mania), normal or decreased, i.e. poverty of speech (dementia, depression, schizophrenia).
- **Tone:** Monotonous (depression) or tremulous (anxiety).
- **Dysarthria** (disorder in articulating speech) and **dysphasia** (disorder in language).

Mood and affect (*Fig. 2.2.1*)

- **Mood** refers to a patient's **sustained, subjective, experienced emotion over a period of time**.
- **Affect** is assessed by observing a patient's **posture, facial expression, emotional reactivity** and **speech**.
- It can be useful to conceptualize the relationship between emotional affect and mood as being similar to that between the weather (**affect**) and the season (**mood**). **Affect** refers to immediate expressions of emotion e.g. smiling at a joke, while **mood** refers to emotional experience over a more prolonged period. Affect is often described as '**reactive**' if no abnormalities are present.
- The patient's mood should be observed throughout the interview with both verbal and non-verbal cues. **Mood** is assessed:

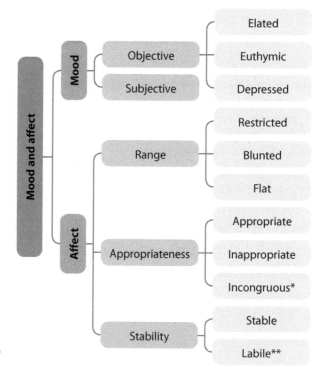

Fig. 2.2.1: Describing mood and affect.
*Incongruous affect: e.g. schizophrenic patient who reports feeling suicidal with a happy facial expression. **Labile mood:** refers to a fluctuating mood state, e.g. that in mania (from elated to euthymic) or delirium.

1. **Objectively** (your impression of their mood): euthymic, elated or depressed.
2. **Subjectively** (the patient's report of their own mood): 'How are you feeling in yourself?', 'How has your mood been lately?'

NOTE: It can be helpful to ask the patient to rate their mood on a scale from 1 to 10 where 1 is 'as low as the patient has ever felt', and 10 is 'as good as the patient has ever felt.'

Thought

One of the first things to do is to assess the patient's way of thinking. Normal human thought has three characteristics: thought content, thought form and thought stream (*Fig. 2.2.2*).

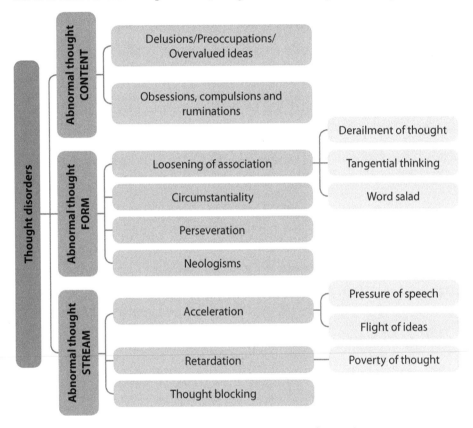

Fig. 2.2.2: Thought divided into abnormalities of thought content, form and stream.

Thought content (*what is being thought about*)

- **Delusions: Fixed false beliefs**, which are **firmly held despite evidence to the contrary** and go **against** the individual's normal **social** and **cultural belief system**. 'Do you have any personal beliefs that others find strange?' See *Fig. 2.2.3* for classification of delusions.
- **Obsessional thoughts: Distressing thoughts** that enter the mind **despite the patient's effort to resist them**. This is a feature of obsessive–compulsive disorder. 'Do certain ideas or images keep entering your mind, even when you try to keep them out?'
- **Preoccupations/overvalued ideas: Strongly held beliefs** which are particularly important in four disorders: depressive, anxiety, eating and sexual. **Preoccupations** differ from obsessions in that they can be put out of the mind with effort, whereas obsessions repeatedly enter the patient's mind despite their attempted resistance.

Classifying delusions

In terms of CAUSE	In association with MOOD	In terms of PLAUSIBILITY	In terms of CONTENT
Primary vs. secondary	Mood congruent vs. mood incongruent	Bizarre vs. non-bizarre	See *Table 2.2.1*

Fig. 2.2.3: There are several ways of classifying delusions. In terms of cause: **primary** is unconnected to previous ideas or events whereas **secondary delusions** arise from, and are understandable in the context of previous ideas or events. **Bizarre delusions** are completely impossible and not in keeping with reality. In **mood congruent delusions**, the content is appropriate to the patient's mood and vice versa in mood incongruent.

Table 2.2.1: Types of delusions in terms of content	
Type of delusion	**Definition (a fixed, false belief that…)**
Grandiose	…one has special powers, is talented, wealthy or important. Grandiose delusions may be religious in nature, e.g. one is chosen by God.
Persecutory	…other people are conspiring against them in order to inflict harm or destroy their reputation.
Reference	…random events, objects or the behaviour of others, have a special significance to oneself.
Guilt	…one has done something sinful or shameful.
Hypochondriacal	…one has a medical illness, despite sound medical evidence to the contrary.
De Clérambault's syndrome (erotomania)	…an exalted person is in love with them. A form of paranoid delusion that is amorous in nature – usually seen in women.
Othello syndrome (morbid jealousy)	…the patient's spouse or sexual partner is being unfaithful without having any actual proof to support their claim.
Capgras' syndrome	…a familiar person or place has been replaced with an exact duplicate – a delusion of misidentification.
Nihilistic (includes Cotard's syndrome)	…they are worthless or dying. In severe cases they claim that everything is non-existent including themselves (*Cotard's syndrome*).
Infestation	…one is infested by small organisms.

Table 2.2.1: Types of delusions in terms of content *(continued)*	
Type of delusion	**Definition**
Folie à deux	A syndrome in which a delusional belief is shared between two people. This is very rare but can occasionally be seen. Often the two people are from the same family.
Delusional memory (rare primary delusion)	Where a delusional belief is based upon the recall of memory or false memory for a past experience. For example, a man recalls seeing a woman giggling at him in a restaurant a couple of weeks ago and now realizes that this person knew he was infested by small organisms.

Thought form (*in what manner, or shape, is the thought brought about*)

Formal thought disorder refers to abnormalities of the way thoughts are linked together:

- Loosening of association: Refers to the loss of the normal structure of thinking. This occurs mainly in schizophrenia. There are three types: (1) **Derailment of thought** (Knight's move thinking): Discourse consisting of a sequence of unrelated or only remotely related ideas. (2) **Tangential thinking:** The person diverts from the original train of thought but never returns to it. It is more indicative of psychopathology as opposed to circumstantiality (*see below*). (3) **Word salad:** Refers to speech that is reduced to a senseless repetition of sounds and phrases.
- Circumstantiality: **Thinking proceeds slowly** with many **unnecessary details** and **digressions**, before **returning to the original point**. This is seen in obsessional personalities and learning disability (LD).
- Neologisms: Are **words and phrases devised by the patient** or a new meaning to an already known word. May be seen in schizophrenia and autism.
- Perseveration: Uncontrollable and inappropriate repetition of a particular response, such as a word, phrase, or gesture. This most often occurs in dementia.

Stream or flow (*the amount and speed of thinking*)

- Acceleration: Accelerated thoughts can manifest as: (1) **Pressured thought**, and (2) **Flight of ideas** – language that may be difficult to understand when it switches quickly from one loosely connected idea to another. These often occur in manic illness.
- Retardation: Slow speed of thinking which occurs in depressive illnesses.
- Thought blocking: Refers to the sudden cessation of flow of thoughts. The previous idea may then be taken up again or replaced by another thought. This mainly occurs in schizophrenia.

Schneider's first rank symptoms (*Table 2.2.2*)

- Screen for schizophrenia by asking about Schneider's first rank symptoms: **Delusional perception**, **third person auditory hallucinations**, **thought interference** (thought insertion, withdrawal and broadcast) and **passivity phenomenon**.

Table 2.2.2: Schneider's first rank symptoms	
Delusional perception	A true perception, to which a patient attributes a false meaning. For example, a perfectly normal event such as the sun coming down may be interpreted by the patient as meaning that he is chosen by God.
Third person auditory hallucination	See *Table 2.2.3* and *OSCE tips 2*.
Thought interference	1. **Thought insertion:** 'Does it feel like your thoughts are your own?' In thought insertion the patient experiences thoughts inside their mind that they identify as not belonging to them, and that have been put there by an external agency. 2. **Thought withdrawal:** 'Does it feel as though your own thoughts are being taken away from you?' 3. **Thought broadcast:** 'Does it feel as though your thoughts are being heard out loud?'
Passivity phenomenon	'Do you ever feel that your mood or actions are being controlled by someone or something else?'

Thoughts of suicide and self-harm

- Ask about **suicidal ideation**: 'Do you think life is worth living?', 'Have things ever got so bad that you have thought of taking your own life?', 'Have you made any plans to end your life?'
- Ask about **self-harm, self-neglect, exploitation of others** and possible **violent** or **homicidal thoughts**. 'Have you had desires to hurt others? If so, in what way?'

Perception

- Determine whether there are any hallucinations. A hallucination is a **perception** in the **absence** of an **external stimulus**. It is a common feature of psychosis.
- Hallucinations may be **visual, auditory, olfactory, gustatory** or **somatic** (*Table 2.2.3*). **Auditory hallucinations** are the **most common** in mental health disorders.
- Hallucinations may be confused with the following:

1. Pseudohallucination: Would include the experience of hearing voices inside your head. They are not true external hallucinations.

2. Illusion: A false mental image produced by misinterpretation of an external stimulus (*Fig. 2.2.4*). Often occurs in normal people.

3. Depersonalization (feature of neurosis): Feeling of detachment from the normal sense of self. 'Do you ever feel unreal or that a part of your body is unreal?'

4. Derealization (feature of neurosis): Feeling of unreality in which the environment and people are experienced as unreal. The patient has got insight and realizes that these experiences are originating from their own mind. 'Do you ever feel that the things around you are unreal?', 'Have you ever had the feeling that things around you are like a stage set?'

Fig. 2.2.4: Illusion of a sleeping baby formed by the clouds.

Table 2.2.3: Screening for hallucinations

Type of hallucination	Definition	How to phrase question NOTE: Prior to asking these questions open with an introductory point, e.g. 'Sometimes when people are distressed they can hear or see things that other people cannot…'
Visual	Seeing things in the absence of an external stimulus, e.g. seeing a unicorn or leprechaun.	'Can you see certain things that others cannot?', 'Do you sometimes see something but when you try to touch it you cannot feel it there?'
Auditory	Hearing sounds or voices in the absence of an external stimulus: **Second person** – voice(s) directly addressing the patient; **Third person** – voices talking amongst themselves, or about the patient; **Running commentary** – voice(s) giving account of what the patient is doing.	'Can you hear things that others cannot?', 'Do the voices sound like normal voices?', 'Can you give me examples of what the voices say?', 'If so, how many voices are there?', 'Do you recognize these voices?', 'When do you hear the voices?', 'Do they speak to you, or about you?', 'Do they comment on what you do?', 'Do the voices tell you to do things?', 'Do you reply to the voices?'
Olfactory	Smelling things in the absence of external stimuli. It is usually an unpleasant smell.	'Have you noticed any unusual smells that you cannot account for and there is nothing to explain them?'
Gustatory	Tasting things in the absence of external stimuli.	'Can you taste things for which there is no explanation?'
Somatic	Abnormal bodily sensations in the absence of external stimuli, e.g. the feeling of insects crawling up the patient's skin.	'Have you noticed any unusual sensations in your body?'

OSCE tips 2: Finding the cause of the hallucination

- **Visual hallucinations** are more characteristic of an organic brain disease or substance misuse (they are rarer in schizophrenia, where auditory hallucinations in the second or third person are more common).
- **Second person auditory hallucinations**, particularly derogatory in nature, are seen in a number of conditions including schizophrenia, severe depression with psychosis and mania with psychosis.
- **Third person auditory hallucinations**, particularly running commentary, is typical of schizophrenia (one of Schneider's first rank symptoms). You do not see third person auditory hallucinations in other psychotic conditions.

Cognition

- **Cognition** consists of **consciousness**, **orientation**, **attention** (ability to focus on the matter at hand), **concentration** (ability to sustain focus) and **memory** (short-term and long-term).
- **Assess general observations:** Are they able to concentrate and make conversation or do they appear confused?
- **Orientation to time**, **place and person**: 'Do you know where we are?', 'Do you remember who I am?', 'Do you know roughly what time it is to the nearest hour?'
- Tools such as the Mini-Mental State Examination **(MMSE)**, the Abbreviated Mental Test **(AMT)**, the Addenbrooke's Cognitive Examination **(ACE)** or the Montreal Cognitive Assessment **(MOCA)** can be helpful in testing memory, attention, language and visuospatial skills (see *Section 10.2*, Dementia).
- **Impaired cognition** is the core feature of organic disorders such as **dementia** and **delirium**.

Insight

- **Insight** is the **extent to which the patient understands the nature of the problem** and if they are in agreement with treatment. Insight can be **intact** (accept that they have mental disorder and are thus willing to accept medication), **partial** (accept that they may have a mental disorder but decline medication, or may deny mental disorder and accept medication) or **non-existent** (categorically deny any mental disorder).
  - 'Do you think you are suffering from a mental illness?'
  - 'If so, would you take medication for it, or let us help you in alternative ways?'
  - 'If we were to give you some medication to help you, would you take it?'

OSCE tips 3: MSE summarized

1. **Appearance** and **behaviour:** Physical state, clothing and accessories, eye contact, facial expression, body language, motor activity, ability to build a rapport.
2. **Speech:** Rate, rhythm, tone, volume, quantity, content.
3. **Mood** and **affect:** Subjective mood (patient's own words), objective mood (euthymic, elated, depressed). Affect (flat, blunted, restricted, appropriate, inappropriate, stable, labile, incongruous).
4. **Thought:** Delusions? Obsessions? Suicidal ideation? Thought interference? Passivity phenomenon? Formal thought disorder?
5. **Perceptions:** Visual, auditory, somatic, gustatory, olfactory hallucinations.
6. **Cognition:** Orientation to time, place and person, memory (MMSE if time permits), concentration and attention.
7. **Insight:** Full, partial, none.

OSCE tips 4: Presenting a mental state examination – an example

I performed a mental state examination on Mr X, aged 35 who is currently unemployed.
I immediately noted that he appeared **unkempt** as I entered the room. Throughout the
examination I noticed he looked **tearful** and had a **downward gaze**, but he was able to build
a rapport with me. His speech seemed **soft and slow in nature** with **poverty of speech**.
Subjectively he describes his mood as **low** and **objectively** he appears **depressed**. His affect
appears to be reactive as he became more tearful when speaking about distressing events.
He does not have formal thought disorder and no disorder of thought stream, or thought
interference. There were no delusions currently present when asked. It is vital to note, however,
that he did have **suicidal ideation** but had no active suicide plans. His wife and kids are
protective factors for him. He also suffers from **second person auditory hallucinations**
which were **derogatory** in nature. There are no abnormal perceptions in any other modalities.
He is oriented to time, place and person though his cognition has not been formally tested.
His **insight is intact** as he feels that he is suffering from depression and feels he requires
medication for this. In conclusion, I think that Mr X is suffering from **severe psychotic
depression with suicidal ideation** and should be referred either informally (if possible)
or on a formal basis (if he refuses) for further assessment and appropriate inpatient treatment.

Chapter 3

Mood disorders

Overview of mood disorders

Definitions

- **Mood:** Refers to a patient's **sustained**, **experienced emotional state** over a period of time. It may be reported **subjectively** (in the patient's own words) or **objectively** as **dysthymic** (low), **euthymic** (normal) or **elated** (elevated).
- **Affect:** Refers to the **transient flow of emotion** in **response to a particular stimulus**. The assessment of mood and affect are described in the *Mental state examination, Section 2.2.*
- Fluctuations in mood are a normal part of human experience. It is only when a disturbance of mood is severe enough to cause **impairment in the activities of daily living** (ADL), that it is considered as a mood disorder.
- **Mood disorder:** Otherwise known as an '**affective disorder**', is any condition characterized by **distorted**, **excessive** or **inappropriate** moods or emotions for a **sustained period of time**.

ICD-10 Classification of affective disorders

1. **Manic episode:** including hypomania, mania without psychotic symptoms and mania with psychotic symptoms.
2. **Bipolar affective disorder.**
3. **Depressive episode:** including mild, moderate, severe and severe with psychotic symptoms.
4. **Recurrent depressive disorder.**
5. **Persistent mood disorders:** cyclothymia, dysthymia.
6. **Other mood disorders.**
7. **Unspecified mood disorder.**

Classification of mood disorders

See *Figs. 3.1.1* and *3.1.2*, and ICD-10 classification.

Mood disorders can be **primary** or **secondary**:

1. **Primary mood disorder:** a mood disorder that does not result from another medical or psychiatric condition. Broadly speaking, a primary mood disorder is either **unipolar** (**depressive disorder**, **dysthymia**) or **bipolar** (**bipolar affective disorder**, **cyclothymia**).
2. **Secondary mood disorder:** a mood disorder that results from another medical or psychiatric condition.

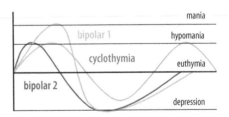

Fig. 3.1.1: Relationship of bipolar 1, bipolar 2 and cyclothymia to mood.

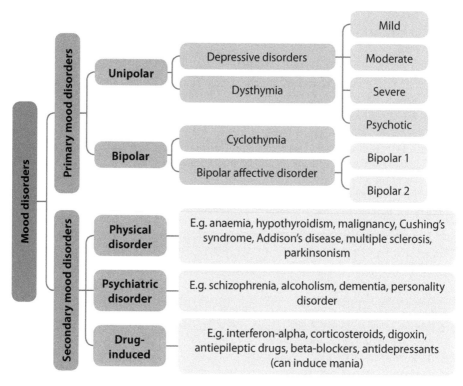

Fig. 3.1.2: Classification of mood disorders.

Depressive disorder is an **affective mood disorder** characterized by a persistent **low mood**, **loss of pleasure** and/or **lack of energy** accompanied by **emotional**, **cognitive** and **biological symptoms**.

Pathophysiology/Aetiology

- Depression is a highly complex **multifactorial disorder** influenced by a number of **bio-psychosocial factors** (see *Table 3.2.1*).
- **Monozygotic twin studies** show the heritability of depression as **40–50%**, and it is likely that multiple genes are involved.
- The **monoamine hypothesis** states that a deficiency of **monoamines (noradrenaline, serotonin and dopamine)** causes depression; this is supported by the fact that antidepressants which increase the concentration of these neurotransmitters in the synaptic cleft, improve the clinical features of depression.
- Over-activity of the **hypothalamic–pituitary–adrenal (HPA) axis** has been linked to depression.
- Psychosocial factors such as **personality type**, **stressful life events** and **failure of effective stress control mechanisms** increase the likelihood of developing depression.

Table 3.2.1: Aetiological factors in depressive disorder

	Biological	Psychological	Social
Predisposing	• Female gender (2:1) • Postnatal period • Genetics: 40–50% monozygotic concordance rates, family history • Neurochemical: ↓ serotonin, ↓ noradrenaline, ↓ dopamine • Endocrine: ↑ activity of HPA axis • Physical co-morbidities • Past history of depression	• Personality type • Failure of effective stress control mechanisms • Poor coping strategies • Other mental health co-morbidities (e.g. dementia)	• Stressful life events • Lack of social support • More common in asylum seeker and refugee population
Precipitating	• Poor compliance with medication • Corticosteroids	• Acute stressful life events (e.g. personal injury, loss of loved one, bankruptcy)	• Unemployment • Poverty • Divorce
Perpetuating	• Chronic health problems (e.g. diabetes, COPD, CCF and chronic pain syndromes)	• Poor insight • Negative thoughts about self, the world and the future (Beck's triad)	• Alcohol and substance misuse • Poor social support • ↓ Social status

Epidemiology and risk factors (see Table 3.2.1)

- Depressive disorders are among the leading causes of disability worldwide. Globally **>350 million** people suffer from depression.
- In General Practice in the UK, each year, about **1 in 20 adults** experience an episode of depression.
- Onset is most commonly in the **40s** (in ♂) and **30s** (in ♀).

> **OSCE tips 1:** Risk factor mnemonic 'FF, AA, PP, SS':
>
> - **F**emale/**F**amily history
> - **A**lcohol/**A**dverse events
> - **P**ast depression/**P**hysical co-morbidities
> - ↓ **S**ocial support/↓ **S**ocioeconomic status

Clinical features

- The symptoms of a depressive disorder can be divided into **core**, **cognitive**, **biological** and **psychotic** (see Table 3.2.2).

> **OSCE tips 2:** A useful mnemonic for the main symptoms of depression - **'DEAD SWAMP'**:
>
> - **D**epressed mood
> - **E**nergy loss (anergia)
> - **A**nhedonia
> - **D**eath thoughts (suicide)
> - **S**leep disturbance
> - **W**orthlessness or guilt
> - **A**ppetite or weight change
> - **M**entation (concentration) reduced
> - **P**sychomotor retardation

Table 3.2.2: Clinical features of depressive disorder	
Core symptoms	
Anhedonia	Lack of interest in things which were previously enjoyable to the patient.
Low mood	Present for at least 2 weeks.
Lack of energy	Also known as anergia.
Cognitive symptoms	
Lack of concentration	Diminished ability to think or concentrate, nearly every day.
Negative thoughts	See Fig. 3.2.1.
Excessive guilt	Feelings of worthlessness or excessive or inappropriate guilt, nearly every day.
Suicidal ideation	Recurrent thoughts of death, recurrent suicidal ideation without a specific plan.
Biological symptoms	
Diurnal variation in mood (DVM)	The patient's low mood is more pronounced during certain times of the day, usually in the morning.
Early morning wakening (EMW)	Waking up to 2 hours earlier than they usually would premorbidly. In atypical depression, there may be hypersomnia (excessive sleep).
Loss of libido	Reduced sexual drive.

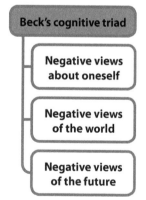

Fig. 3.2.1: **Beck's cognitive triad** represents three types of negative thought. The triad involves negative thoughts about: the self (i.e. the patient feels worthless), the world/environment (i.e. the world is unfair), and the future (i.e. the future is hopeless).

Table 3.2.2: Clinical features of depressive disorder *(continued)*	
Biological symptoms	
Psychomotor retardation	Refers to slow speech as well as slow movement.
Weight loss and loss of appetite	Significant weight loss when not dieting, or decrease in appetite nearly every day. Weight gain and increased appetite may occur in atypical depression.
Psychotic symptoms	
Hallucinations	These are usually second person auditory hallucinations.
Delusions	These are usually hypochondriacal, guilt, nihilistic or persecutory in nature.

ICD-10 Classification of depression

Mild depression = **2** *core* symptoms + **2** *other* symptoms
Moderate depression = **2** *core* symptoms + **3–4** *other* symptoms
Severe depression = **3** *core* symptoms + **≥4** *other* symptoms
Severe depression with psychosis = **3** *core* symptoms + **≥4** *other* symptoms + *psychosis*

Diagnosis and investigations

Hx
- **Explore the core symptoms:** 'How has your mood been recently?' **(low mood)**, 'Do you still enjoy the things that you used to?' **(anhedonia)**, 'Do you find yourself feeling tired more easily or more worn out?' **(anergia)**
- **Explore the cognitive symptoms:** 'Are you able to concentrate on activities, for example, watching a television programme?' **(lack of concentration)**, 'How do you see things unfolding in the future?' **(negative thoughts)**, 'Do you feel life is worth living?', 'Have you had any thoughts of taking your own life?' **(suicidal)***
- **Explore the biological symptoms:** 'Do you find your mood particularly worse during certain times of the day?' **(DVM)**, 'What time did you used to wake up before you felt low in mood?', 'What time do you wake up now?' **(EMW)**, 'Has anyone around you mentioned that you seem low or restless?' **(psychomotor retardation)**, 'When people feel down, sometimes their sexual drive also goes down, has this happened to you?' **(loss of libido)**

*If the patient suggests that they are actively suicidal, you must carry out a full risk assessment (see Suicide and risk assessment, *Section 9.2*).

OSCE tips 3: DO NOT forget to rule out important differential diagnoses!

Remember to always consider other important differential diagnoses even when the symptoms described are very typical of depression. Always ask yourself, 'Is there another psychiatric condition to consider?' e.g. bipolar affective disorder (i.e. did the patient ever have an excessive elevation of mood in the past?). 'Have I ruled out **organic illnesses** that can present with depression?' e.g. thyroid dysfunction.

MSE	Appearance	Signs of self-neglect, thin, unkempt, depressed facial expression, tearful.
	Behaviour	Poor eye contact, tearful, psychomotor retardation, slow movements, slow responses, may sometimes present with psychomotor agitation.
	Speech	May be slow, non-spontaneous, reduced volume and tone.
	Mood	Low (subjectively) and depressed (objectively).
	Thought	Pessimistic, guilty, worthless, helpless, suicidal, delusions (if psychotic).
	Perception	Second person auditory hallucinations (often derogatory).
	Cognition	Impaired concentration.
	Insight	Usually good.

Ix

Investigations are used to exclude organic causes for depression. They are not mandatory and should be used according to clinical judgement:

- **Diagnostic questionnaires:** e.g. **PHQ-9**, **HADS** and **Beck's depression inventory**.
- **Blood tests: FBC** (e.g. to check for anaemia), **TFTs** (e.g. to test for hypothyroidism), **U&Es**, **LFTs**, **calcium levels** (biochemical abnormalities may cause physical symptoms which can mimic some depressive symptoms), **glucose** (diabetes can cause anergia).
- **Imaging: MRI** or **CT scan** may be required where presentation or examination is atypical or where there are features suspicious of an intracranial lesion e.g. unexplained headache or personality change.

DDx

- **Other mood disorders:** Bipolar affective disorder, other depressive disorders (see *Key facts 1*).
- **Secondary to physical condition** e.g. hypothyroidism (see Overview of mood disorders, *Section 3.1*).
- **Secondary to psychoactive substance abuse.**
- **Secondary to other psychiatric disorders:** Psychotic disorders, anxiety disorders, adjustment disorder, personality disorder, eating disorders, dementia.
- **Normal bereavement.**

Key facts 1: Other depressive disorders

- **Recurrent depressive disorder:** A recurrent depressive episode refers to when a patient has another depressive episode after their first.
- **Seasonal affective disorder:** Characterized by depressive episodes recurring annually at the same time each year, usually during the winter months.
- **Masked depression:** A state in which depressed mood is not particularly prominent, but other features of a depressive disorder are, e.g. sleep disturbance, diurnal variation in mood.
- **Atypical depression:** This typically occurs with mild–moderate depression with reversal of symptoms e.g. overeating, weight gain and hypersomnia. There is a relationship between atypical depression and seasonal affective disorder.
- **Dysthymia:** Depressive state for at least 2 years, which does not meet the criteria for a mild, moderate or severe depressive disorder and is not the result of a partially-treated depressive illness.
- **Cyclothymia:** Chronic mood fluctuation over at least a 2-year period with episodes of elation and of depression which are insufficient to meet the criteria for a hypomanic or a depressive disorder.
- **Baby blues:** Seen in around 60–70% of women, typically 3–7 days following birth, and is more common in primiparae. Mothers are anxious, tearful and irritable. Reassurance and support is all that is required.
- **Postnatal depression:** Affects approximately 10% of women. Most cases start within a month and typically peak at 3 months. Clinical features are similar to depression seen in other circumstances.

Management (includes NICE guidance 2009)

- The broad treatment of depression is highlighted using the **bio-psychosocial approach** (*Fig. 3.2.2*).
- The management of depression depends on the **severity** of the depression.

Management of mild–moderate depression (NICE guidelines 2009)

- **Watchful waiting:** Should be considered and reassess the patient again in **2 weeks**.
- **Antidepressants: Not** recommended as a first-line therapy for mild depression unless: (1) depression has **lasted a long time**; (2) **past history** of **moderate–severe** depression; (3) **failure of other interventions**; (4) or the depression **complicates the care of other physical health problems**.
- **Self-help programmes:** Patient works through a **self-help manual** with a healthcare professional providing support and checking progress.
- **Computerized cognitive behavioural therapy (CBT):** Based on **conventional CBT**, involves a **computer programme** educating them about depression and challenging negative thoughts.

Biological
• **Antidepressants**
• **Adjuvants** e.g. antipsychotics
• **Electroconvulsive therapy**

Psychological
• **Psychotherapies** (See *Key facts 2*)
• **Self-help programmes**
• **Physical activity**

Social
• **Social support groups**

Fig. 3.2.2: Bio-psychosocial approach to depression.

- **Physical activity programme:** Exercise has been shown to benefit mental health. **Group exercise class** under the supervision of a qualified trainer may be recommended.
- **Psychotherapies** (see *Key facts 2*): If the options above fail, psychotherapies can be tried.

Management of moderate–severe depression (*NICE guidelines 2009*)

- **Suicide risk assessment:** Should be performed on all patients.
- **Psychiatry referral:** Indicated if: (1) **suicide risk** is **high**; (2) depression is **severe**; (3) **recurrent** depression; (4) or **unresponsive** to **initial treatment**.
- **Mental Health Act:** Implementation may become necessary in some cases.
- **Antidepressants: First-line** antidepressants are **selective serotonin reuptake inhibitors** (SSRIs) e.g. citalopram. Other antidepressants include **tricyclic antidepressants (TCAs)**, **serotonin noradrenaline reuptake inhibitors (SNRIs)** and **monoamine oxidase inhibitors** (MAOIs can only be prescribed by specialists). Should be **continued for 6 months** after resolution of symptoms for first depressive episode, 2 years after resolution of second episode, and long term in individuals who have had multiple severe episodes.
- **Adjuvants:** Antidepressants may be **augmented** with **lithium**, or **antipsychotics**.
- **Psychotherapy:** Refer for **CBT** and **interpersonal therapy (IPT)**.
- **Social support:** Engaging with activities in the community that the individual is avoiding or attending social support groups with others.
- **ECT:** Indications specific to depression include: (1) acute treatment of **severe depression** which is **life-threatening**; (2) **rapid response required**; (3) **depression** with **psychotic features**; (4) **severe psychomotor retardation** or **stupor**; (5) or **failure of other treatments**.

Key facts 2: Psychotherapies used to manage depression (see *Section 12.1*, Psychotherapies)

- **CBT:** Depression causes negative thoughts, which can lead to negative behaviours. CBT allows people to identify and tackle negative thoughts; conducted in groups or individually.
- **IPT:** Helps to identify and solve relationship problems, whether it is with family, partners or friends.
- **Behavioural activation:** Encourages depressed patients to develop more positive behaviour or activities that they would usually avoid.
- **Counselling:** Enables patients to explore their problems and symptoms. Counsellors offer support and guide patients to help themselves for a particular focus, e.g. bereavement or relationship counselling.
- **Psychodynamic therapy:** Aim is to explore and understand the dynamics and difficulties of a patient's life, which may have begun in childhood.

Self-assessment

A 45-year-old woman presents with a one-month history of low mood, lack of energy and weight loss, in the setting of a recent divorce. She explains an inability to keep her concentration focused on work and expresses feelings of worthlessness and hopelessness. You suspect depression.

1. Two of the three core symptoms of depression have been mentioned, what is the third? *(1 mark)*

2. What is the severity of her depression? *(1 mark)*

3. What are the biological symptoms of depression? *(4 marks)*

4. Which organic cause of depression must you rule out and what blood test must be ordered to test this? *(2 marks)*

5. You determine the patient to be suffering from severe depression. What is the first-line pharmacological treatment of moderate–severe depression? Give an example of a drug that falls in this group. *(2 marks)*

6. Give three indications for the use of ECT in the management of depression. *(3 marks)*

Answers to self-assessment questions are to be found in *Appendix B*.

3.3 Bipolar affective disorder

Definition

Bipolar affective disorder (previously known as '**manic depression**') is a **chronic episodic mood disorder**, characterized by at least one episode of **mania** (or **hypomania**) and a further episode of mania or depression. Either one can occur first but the term bipolar also includes those who at the time of diagnosis have suffered only manic episodes, as all cases of mania will eventually develop depression.

Pathophysiology/Aetiology

- The cause of bipolar affective disorder (BPAD) involves both **biological** and **environmental** factors (*Fig. 3.3.1*).
- The **monoamine hypothesis** is applicable to elevated mood just as it is to depressed mood. It states that elevated mood is a result of **increased central monoamines** (**noradrenaline** and **serotonin**).
- **Dysfunction of the HPA axis** (abnormal secretion of cortisol, as found in unipolar depression) and dysfunction of the hypothalamic–pituitary–thyroid axis may contribute to BPAD.
- BPAD shows **strong heritability** with **monozygotic twin studies** showing a **40–70%** concordance rate. The lifetime risk of developing BPAD for 1st degree relatives of a BPAD patient is **5–10%**.
- **Stressful** or **significant life events** may precipitate the onset of a first manic episode.

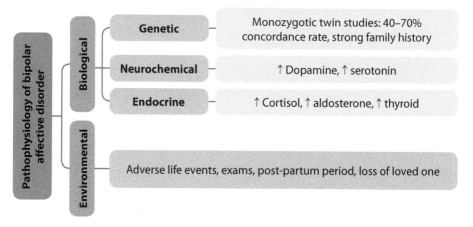

Fig. 3.3.1: Outline of the biological and environmental factors associated with BPAD.

Epidemiology and risk factors (*Table 3.3.1*)

- The lifetime risk of developing BPAD is **1–3%**.
- The mean age of onset is **19** years of age.
- In the UK, the incidence of bipolar disorder is higher in **black** and other **minority ethnic groups** than in the white population.
- The male to female affected ratio is **1:1**.

Table 3.3.1: Risk factors for bipolar affective disorder (Aggressive Spenders)	
Age in early-20's	Strong Family Hx
Anxiety disorders	Substance misuse
After depression	Stressful life events

Clinical features

- The symptoms of BPAD include those of mania or depression. Manic symptoms are listed in *Table 3.3.2* and the symptoms of depression have been discussed in *Section 3.2*, Depressive disorder.
- The severity of mania can be divided into: (1) **hypomania**; (2) **mania without psychosis**; (3) and **mania with psychosis** depending on the severity of symptoms (*Fig. 3.3.2*).
- Different types of bipolar disorder have been recognized according to DSM-V (*Table 3.3.3*).

Table 3.3.2: Symptoms of mania 'DIG FASTER'

Irritability	**A**ctivity/**A**ppetite increased
Distractibility/**D**isinhibited (sexual, social, spending)	**S**leep decreased
Insight impaired/**I**ncreased libido	**T**alkative – pressure of speech
Grandiose delusions	**E**levated mood/**E**nergy increased
Flight of ideas	**R**educed concentration/**R**eckless behaviour and spending

Hypomania	Mania without psychosis	Mania with psychosis
• **Mildly elevated mood** or **irritable mood** present for **≥4 days**. Symptoms of mania, where present, are to a **lesser extent** than true mania. Considerable interference with work and social life but **not severe disruption**. **Partial insight** may be preserved.	• As with hypomania but to a **greater extent**. Symptoms present for **>1 week**, with **complete disruption** of work and social activities. May have **grandiose ideas** and excessive spending could lead to debts. There may be **sexual disinhibition** and reduced sleep may lead to **exhaustion**.	• **Severely elevated** or **suspicious mood** with the addition of psychotic features such as **grandiose** or **persecutory delusions** and **auditory hallucinations** that are mood congruent. Patient may show signs of **aggression**.

Fig. 3.3.2: Summary of manic mood disorders that contribute to bipolar affective disorder.

Table 3.3.3: Classification of bipolar affective disorder

Bipolar I	Bipolar II	Rapid cycling
Involves periods of severe mood episodes from mania to depression.	Milder form of mood elevation, involving milder episodes of hypomania that alternate with periods of severe depression.	More than four mood swings in a 12-month period with no intervening asymptomatic periods. Poor prognosis.

ICD-10 Criteria for mania and bipolar affective disorder

Mania requires **3/9** symptoms to be present: (1) Grandiosity/inflated self-esteem; (2) Decreased sleep; (3) Pressure of speech; (4) Flight of ideas; (5) Distractibility; (6) Psychomotor agitation (restlessness); (7) Reckless behaviour, e.g. spending sprees, reckless driving; (8) Loss of social inhibitions (leading to inappropriate behaviour); (9) Marked sexual energy.

- **Bipolar affective disorder** requires at least **two** episodes in which a person's mood and activity levels are significantly disturbed – **one** of which MUST be **mania** or **hypomania**.
- ICD-10 divides bipolar disorder into **five states**: (1) Currently hypomanic; (2) Currently manic; (3) Currently depressed; (4) Mixed Disorder; (5) In remission.

Diagnosis and investigations

Hx
- 'How would you describe your mood?' **(elevated, depressed or irritable mood)**.
- 'Have you ever felt on top of the world?' **(elevated mood)**.
- 'Do you feel that you have too much energy compared to those around you?' **(↑ energy)**.
- 'Are you able to concentrate on routine activities?' **(↓ concentration)**.
- 'Do you find yourself needing less sleep but not getting tired?' **(↓ sleep and ↑ energy levels)**.
- 'Has your interest in sex changed?' **(↑ libido)**.
- 'Have you had any new interests or exciting ideas lately?' **(delusions/overvalued ideas)**.
- 'Do you have any special abilities that are unique to you?' **(grandiose delusions)**.
- 'Are you afraid that someone is trying to harm you?' **(persecutory delusions)**.
- Also ask about **family history** of bipolar affective disorder and **substance misuse**.
- **Pressure of speech** and **flight of ideas** can be assessed from the conversation.

OSCE tips 1: Remember to always screen for mania in a depressed patient!

- A patient may present with the classic symptoms of depression but may actually be suffering from bipolar.
- They may not initially reveal to you that they have previously had a manic episode(s) so it is very important that you specifically ask whether they have had previous instances where their mood has been significantly elevated. Also ask about previous periods of over-activity or disinhibition.
- Be vigilant. Do not fall into the trap of diagnosing depressive disorder immediately, otherwise your diagnosis will be incorrect and subsequently your management will go down the wrong path – with adverse consequences.

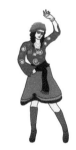

Fig. 3.3.3: Individual with inappropriate bright clothing in keeping with possible mania.

MSE	Appearance	Flamboyant/unusual combination of clothing (see *Fig. 3.3.3*), heavy makeup and jewellery. Personal neglect when condition is severe.
	Behaviour	Overfamiliar, disinhibited (flirtatious, aggressive), increased psychomotor activity, distractible, restless.
	Speech	Loud, ↑ rate and quantity, pressure of speech, uninterruptible, puns and rhymes, neologisms.
	Mood	Elated, euphoric, and/or irritable.
	Thought	Optimistic, pressured thought, flight of ideas, loosening of association, circumstantiality, tangentiality, overvalued ideas, grandiose/persecutory delusions.
	Perception	Usually no hallucinations. Mood-congruent auditory hallucinations may occur.
	Cognition	Attention and concentration often impaired. Fully oriented.
	Insight	Generally very poor.

OSCE tips 2: The challenge of history taking in a manic patient

- Eliciting a thorough history from a manic patient is a true test of your communication skills as the task is made difficult by their irritability (80% of manic patients), distractibility and disinhibition.
- Be polite but firm in your approach. Flight of ideas, circumstantiality and tangentiality may cause patients to veer off topic, so the key is to gently redirect the patient back to the asked question.
- Any OSCE station will be time-limited so you will need to take control of the interview to ensure that you ask appropriate questions in order to make a clear diagnosis.

Ix
- **Self-rating scales:** e.g. Mood Disorder Questionnaire.
- **Blood tests: FBC** (routine), **TFTs** (both hyper/hypothyroidism are differentials), **U&Es** (baseline renal function with view to starting lithium), **LFTs** (baseline hepatic function with view to starting mood stabilizers), **glucose**, **calcium** (biochemical disturbances can cause mood symptoms).
- **Urine drug test: Illicit drugs** can cause manic symptoms.
- **CT head:** to rule out space-occupying lesions (can cause manic symptoms such as disinhibition).

- **Mood disorders:** hypomania, mania, mixed episode, cyclothymia.
- **Psychotic disorders:** schizophrenia, schizoaffective disorder.
- **Secondary to medical condition:** hyper/hypothyroidism, Cushing's disease, cerebral tumour (e.g. frontal lobe lesion with disinhibition), stroke.
- **Drug related:** illicit drug ingestion (e.g. amphetamines, cocaine), acute drug withdrawal, side effect of corticosteroid use.
- **Personality disorders:** histrionic, emotionally unstable.

Management (including NICE guidance 2014)

- Full **risk assessment** is vital including suicidal ideation and risk to self (e.g. financial ruin from overspending). This will determine the urgency of referral to specialist mental health services.
- Remember to **ask about driving**. The **DVLA** has clear guidelines about driving when manic, hypomanic or severely depressed.
- The **Mental Health Act** is needed if the patient is violent or a risk to self. **Hospitalization** will be required if there is: (1) **reckless behaviour** causing **risk to patient or others**; (2) significant **psychotic symptoms**; (3) **impaired judgement**; (4) or **psychomotor agitation**.
- The pharmacological management of bipolar affective disorder is shown in *Table 3.3.4*. Also see *Section 12.4*, Mood stabilizers.
- For **bipolar depression**, offer a **high-intensity psychological intervention** (e.g. **CBT**).
- **ECT** is not first-line, but it can be used when antipsychotic drugs are ineffective and the patient is so severely disturbed that further medication or awaiting natural recovery is not feasible.
- Patients who present with an acute episode should be followed-up **once a week initially** and then **2–4 weekly** for the first few months.
- The **bio-psychosocial approach** to BPAD is shown in *Fig. 3.3.4*.

Biological
• **Mood stabilizers**, **benzodiazepines**, **antipsychotics**
• **ECT:** for severe uncontrolled mania

Psychological
• **Psychoeducation**
• **CBT**

Social
• **Social support groups**
• **Self-help groups**
• **Encourage calming activities**

Fig. 3.3.4: Bio-psychosocial approach to the management of BPAD.

OSCE tips 3: A useful mnemonic for the management of bipolar affective disorder: **'CALMER'**

- Consider hospitalization/CBT
- Antipsychotics (Atypical)
- Lorazepam
- Mood stabilizers (e.g. lithium)
- Electroconvulsive therapy
- Risk assessment

Table 3.3.4: Pharmacological management of BPAD

Acute manic episode/mixed episode	Bipolar depressive episode
• First-line: **offer an antipsychotic** such as **olanzapine, risperidone** or **quetiapine** (**haloperidol** is also effective). They have a rapid onset of action compared to mood stabilizers and are therefore used in severe mania. If the first antipsychotic is not effective or poorly tolerated then a second is usually offered. • **Mood stabilizers** namely lithium or if not suitable, valproate should be added as second-line treatment (see Mood stabilizers, *Section 12.4*). • **Benzodiazepines** may further be required to aid sleep and reduce agitation. • **Rapid tranquilization** may be required with **haloperidol** and/or **lorazepam**.	• **Atypical antipsychotics** are effective in bipolar depression. Options include **olanzapine** (combined with **fluoxetine**), **olanzapine alone** or **quetiapine alone**. • **Mood stabilizer** option is **lamotrigine**. Lithium is also effective. • **Antidepressants** alone are usually avoided – if used, they should be used with care in BPAD, even if depression is the main feature, as they have the potential to induce mania. They should be prescribed in conjunction with the cover of anti-manic medication.

Long-term management of bipolar affective disorder

- 4 weeks after an acute episode has resolved, **lithium** should be offered first-line to prevent relapses.
- If lithium is ineffective consider adding **valproate**. **Olanzapine** or **quetiapine** are alternative options.

Key facts: The use of lithium as prophylaxis

- Lithium is the standard **long-term therapy** in bipolar affective disorder. It minimizes the risk of relapse and improves quality of life.
- Before lithium treatment is started **U&Es** (lithium has renal excretion), **TFTs**, **pregnancy status** and baseline **ECG** should be checked. Lithium has a **narrow therapeutic window** and so drug levels should be closely monitored and patients should be informed of potential side effects and toxicity.
- **Side effects** include: polydipsia, polyuria, *fine* tremor, weight gain, oedema, hypothyroidism, impaired renal function, memory problems and teratogenicity (in 1st trimester).
- Signs of **toxicity (1.5–2.0 mmol/L)**: N+V, *coarse* tremor, ataxia, muscle weakness, apathy.
- Signs of **severe toxicity (>2.0 mmol/L)**: nystagmus, dysarthria, hyperreflexia, oliguria, hypotension, convulsions and coma.
- Due to its side effect profile and risk of toxicity lithium is **strictly regulated**:
  - **Lithium levels – 12 hours** following first dose, then **weekly** until **therapeutic level (0.5–1.0 mmol/L)** has been stable for **4 weeks**. Once stable check every **3 months**.
  - **U&Es** – every **6 months**; TFTs – every **12 months**.
- A combination of **lithium and sodium valproate** is first-line treatment for **rapid cycling**.

Self-assessment

A 21-year-old female presents with low mood and anhedonia. She is unemployed and lives with her mother following her father's death in a tragic car accident when she was a young girl. You suspect depression and start her on citalopram. A week later her distressed mother comes to see you as she suspects her daughter has not told you the full story. She mentions that there are periods when her daughter seems full of herself, talks constantly without pausing and acts recklessly (e.g. overspending resulting in the family being in debt). She is also concerned about her daughter's alcohol consumption.

1. What is the most likely diagnosis? *(1 mark)*
2. Give six differential diagnoses. *(3 marks)*
3. Based on the ICD-10 criteria, give three of the nine possible symptoms required to confirm an episode of mania. *(3 marks)*
4. What is the difference between hypomania and mania? *(2 marks)*
5. Name two mood stabilizers that could be offered to a patient with an acute manic episode. What needs to be taken into consideration for a woman this age? *(4 marks)*

Answers to self-assessment questions are to be found in *Appendix B*.

Chapter 4

Psychotic disorders

Definition, classification and epidemiology of psychosis

- **Psychosis** is defined as a mental state in which **reality is greatly distorted**. It typically presents with:

  1. Delusions: A **fixed false belief**, which is **firmly held** despite evidence to the contrary and goes against the individual's **normal social and cultural belief system**. See MSE, Section 2.2 for classification and types of delusions.

  2. Hallucinations: A **perception** in the **absence** of an **external stimulus**. It is a common feature of psychosis. See MSE, Section 2.2 for types of hallucinations.

ICD-10 Classification of schizophrenia and other psychotic disorders

1. **Schizophrenia**
2. **Schizotypal disorder**
3. **Persistent delusional disorder**
4. **Acute and transient psychotic disorders**
5. **Induced delusional disorder**
6. **Schizoaffective disorder**
7. **Other non-organic psychotic disorders**
8. **Unspecified non-organic psychosis**

  3. Thought disorder: An impairment in the ability to form thoughts from logically connected ideas. See MSE, Section 2.2.

- Psychotic disorders are relatively common, with **schizophrenia** being the **most common**.
- The **incidence** of psychosis in England is roughly **31.7 per 100 000** people.
- UK studies suggest a possible **higher prevalence** of psychosis in the **black** and **ethnic minority** populations compared to the white population.
- There are a variety of conditions that can present with **psychosis** (Fig. 4.1.1).
- **Non-organic** causes of psychosis other than schizophrenia are covered in Table 4.1.1.

Causes of psychosis

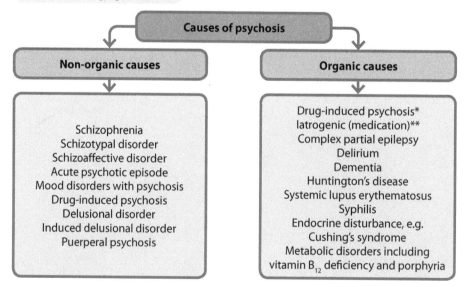

Fig. 4.1.1: Organic and non-organic causes of psychosis.
*Alcohol, cocaine, amphetamine, methamphetamine, methylenedioxy-methamphetamine (MDMA), mephedrone, cannabis, LSD, psilocybins (e.g. magic mushrooms), ketamine; **levodopa, methyldopa, steroids, antimalarials.

Table 4.1.1: Other causes of psychosis
('schizophrenia and schizoaffective persist for >1 month, paraphrenia presents late')

Schizotypal disorder	Also known as **latent schizophrenia**, it is characterized by **eccentric behaviour, suspiciousness, unusual speech** and **deviations of thinking** and **affect** that is similar to those suffering from schizophrenia. These individuals however, **do not** suffer from **hallucinations** or **delusions**. There is an increased risk of schizotypal disorder in those who have first-degree relatives with schizophrenia.
Acute and transient psychotic disorders	A psychotic episode presenting very similarly to schizophrenia but lasting **<1 month** and so not meeting the criteria for schizophrenia.
Schizoaffective disorder	Characterized by both symptoms of **schizophrenia and a mood disorder** (depression or mania) in the **same episode of illness**. The mood symptoms should meet the criteria for either a depressive illness or a manic episode together with one or two typical symptoms of schizophrenia.
Persistent delusional disorder	The development of a **single or set of delusions** for a period of at least **3 months** in which the delusion is the only, or the most prominent, symptom with other areas of thinking and functioning well preserved, unlike in schizophrenia. The content of the delusion is often **persecutory**, **grandiose** or **hypochondriacal** in nature. The onset and content of the delusion is often related to the patient's life situation. Symptoms often respond well to antipsychotics.
Induced delusional disorder (Folie à deux)	Induced delusional disorder, also known as '**shared paranoid disorder**', is an uncommon disorder characterized by the presence of similar delusions in two or more individuals. **Folie imposée** is where a dominant person ('primary') initially forms a delusional belief during a psychotic episode and imposes it on another person(s) ('secondary'). **Folie simultanée** is when two people considered to suffer independently from psychosis, influence the content of each other's delusions so that they become identical or very similar.
Mood disorders with psychosis	Psychosis occurs **secondary to depression or mania**. On the other hand, schizophrenia usually develops spontaneously.
Puerperal Psychosis (or post-partum psychosis)	The **acute onset** of a **manic** or **psychotic episode** shortly after childbirth (usually develops **in the first 2 weeks** following birth). It affects approximately **0.2%** of women.
Late paraphrenia	A term that is sometimes used to describe **late-onset schizophrenia**. It is not coded for in ICD-10. Hallucinations and delusions (particularly paranoid) are prominent, whereas thought disorders and catatonic symptoms are rare.

Schizophrenia

Schizophrenia is the most common **psychotic condition**, characterized by **hallucinations**, **delusions** and **thought disorders** which lead to **functional impairment**. It occurs in the absence of organic disease, alcohol or drug-related disorders and is not secondary to elevation or depression of mood.

Pathophysiology/Aetiology (see Table 4.2.1)

- The aetiology of schizophrenia involves both **biological** and **environmental factors**.
- There is an increased likelihood of schizophrenia in those with a **positive family history**, and **monozygotic twin studies** show a **48%** concordance rate.
- The **dopamine hypothesis** states that schizophrenia is secondary to **over-activity** of **mesolimbic dopamine pathways** in the brain. This is supported by conventional antipsychotics which work by blocking dopamine (D2) receptors, and by drugs that potentiate the pathway (e.g. anti-parkinsonian drugs and amphetamines) causing psychotic symptoms.
- Factors that interfere with early neurodevelopment such as **obstetric complications**, **fetal injury** and **low birth weight** lead to abnormalities expressed in the mature brain.
- **Adverse life events** and **psychological stress** increase the likelihood of developing schizophrenia.
- **Expressed emotion** is the theory that those with relatives that are 'over' involved or that make hostile or excessive critical comments are more likely to relapse.
- The **stress–vulnerability model** predicts that schizophrenia occurs due to environmental factors interacting with a genetic predisposition (or brain injury). Patients have different vulnerabilities and so different individuals need to be exposed to different levels of environmental factors to become psychotic.

Epidemiology and risk factors (see Table 4.2.1)

Table 4.2.1: Aetiological factors in schizophrenia

	Biological	Psychological	Social
Predisposing	• **Genetic:** Monozygotic twin studies – 48% concordance • **Neurochemical:** ↑dopamine, ↓glutamate, ↓serotonin, ↓GABA • **Neurodevelopmental:** Intrauterine infection, premature birth, fetal brain injury and obstetric complications • Age 15–35 • Extremes of parental age: ≤20 years or ≥35 years	• **Family history:** The closer the family relationship to an affected relative, the higher the risk • **Childhood abuse**	• **Substance misuse** • **Low socioeconomic status** • **Migrants:** Higher incidence in migrant populations (e.g. African-Caribbean), but not in offspring born in the new location • Living in an urban area – although this could be as a result of urban drift into cities. • Birth in late winter/early spring season (controversial)

Table 4.2.1: Aetiological factors in schizophrenia *(continued)*			
	Biological	**Psychological**	**Social**
Precipitating	• **Smoking cannabis** or using **psychostimulants**	• Adverse life events • Poor coping style	• Adverse life events
Perpetuating	• Substance misuse • Poor compliance to medication	• Adverse life events	• ↓ Social support • Expressed emotion

- Schizophrenia affects approximately **24 million** people worldwide. The incidence of schizophrenia is estimated to be **5 per 100 000** people.
- Peak age of onset is **15–35 years**.
- **Males** and **females** are **equally** affected but a systematic review showed men aged <45 years had twice the rate of schizophrenia as women.

Clinical features

- The symptoms of schizophrenia can be referred to as positive (the **acute** syndrome) when there is the appearance of hallucinations and delusions. This is in contrast to **negative** symptoms (the **chronic** syndrome) which refers to loss of function. The clinical features of schizophrenia depend upon the type of schizophrenia, with **paranoid schizophrenia** being the most common (*Fig. 4.2.1*).

Positive symptoms (**D**elusions **H**eld **F**irmly **T**hink **P**sychosis)

- **Delusions:** A delusion is a **fixed false belief**, which is **firmly held** despite evidence to the contrary and goes **against** the individual's **normal social** and **cultural belief system**. Usually **persecutory, grandiose, nihilistic,** or **religious** in nature. **Ideas of reference** are thoughts in which a patient infers that common events refer to them directly (e.g. personal messages from television and newspapers).

- **Hallucinations:** A hallucination is a **perception** in the **absence** of an **external stimulus**. They are usually **third person auditory hallucinations** which may be of running commentary nature.

- **Formal thought disorder:** Abnormalities of the way thoughts are linked together. See *Section 2.1*, MSE.

- **Thought interference:** This could either be the feelings that thoughts are being inserted (**thought insertion**), removed (**thought withdrawal**) or heard out loud by others (**thought broadcast**).

- **Passivity phenomenon:** **Actions**, **feelings** or **emotions** being controlled by an external force.

> **Key facts 1:** Schneider's first rank symptoms
>
> **Schneider's first-rank symptoms** of schizophrenia are symptoms which, if one or more are present, are strongly suggestive of schizophrenia and is an **alternative tool to ICD-10** in diagnosing schizophrenia:
> - **Delusional perception:** A new delusion that forms in response to a real perception without any logical sense, e.g. 'the traffic light turned red so I am the chosen one.'
> - **Third person auditory hallucinations:** usually a running commentary.
> - **Thought interference:** thought insertion, withdrawal or broadcast.
> - **Passivity phenomenon.**

Negative symptoms (the **A** factor)

- Avolition (↓ **motivation**): Reduced ability (or inability) to initiate and persist in goal-directed behaviour.
- Asocial behaviour: Loss of drive for any social engagements.
- Anhedonia: Lack of pleasure in activities that were previously enjoyable to the patient.
- Alogia (poverty of speech): A quantitative and qualitative decrease in speech.
- Affect blunted: Diminished or absent capacity to express feelings.
- Attention (cognitive) deficits: May experience problems with attention, language, memory, and executive function.

NOTE: The onset of clinical features may be preceded by a **prodrome** where the patient becomes **reserved**, **anxious**, **suspicious** and **irritable** with a disturbance in normal everyday functioning.

Paranoid schizophrenia

- Most common. Dominated by **positive symptoms** (hallucinations and delusions).

Postschizophrenic depression

- Depression predominates with schizophrenic illness in the past 12 months with some schizophrenia symptoms still present.

Hebephrenic schizophrenia

- **Thought disorganization** predominates. Onset of illness is earlier (15–25) and has poorer prognosis.

Catatonic schizophrenia

- Rare form characterized by one or more **catatonic symptoms**.

Simple schizophrenia

- Rare form where negative symptoms develop without psychotic symptoms.

Undifferentiated schizophrenia

- Meets diagnostic criteria for schizophrenia but does not conform to any of the other subtypes.

Residual schizophrenia

- 1 year of chronic **negative symptoms** preceded by a clear-cut psychotic episode.

Fig. 4.2.1: Classification of schizophrenia according to ICD-10. [*Mnemonic*] **P**aranoid **P**sychotic **H**umans **C**an't **S**upply **U**nderstandable **R**easoning.

ICD-10 Criteria for schizophrenia	
Group A	**Group B**
A. Thought echo/insertion/withdrawal/ broadcast. B. Delusions of control, influence or passivity phenomenon. C. Running commentary auditory hallucinations. D. Bizarre persistent delusions.	E. Hallucinations in other modalities that are persistent. F. Thought disorganization (loosening of associations, neologisms, incoherence). G. Catatonic symptoms. H. Negative symptoms.

At least **one** very clear symptom from **Group A** (A–D) or **two** or more from **Group B** (E–H) for at least **1 month** or more. Schizophrenia should not be diagnosed in the presence of organic brain disease.

OSCE tips: History taking from psychotic patients

- The most common OSCE scenario will be a patient with paranoid schizophrenia displaying positive and perhaps negative symptoms. The other types of schizophrenia are much less common.
- History taking will require you to be familiar with, and look comfortable and confident, asking questions to elicit psychotic symptoms. For the patient their psychotic experiences are real, and you need to demonstrate an empathetic and supportive approach to history taking and MSE.
- Remember to consider the other differentials, both organic and psychiatric, including mood disorders, and drug-induced psychosis.
- A good social history focusing on day to day activities and interests may help you to elicit negative symptoms of schizophrenia.
- You need to sensitively ask questions about insight and risk, as this will determine your management.

Diagnosis and investigations

Hx
- 'Have you ever had the experience of hearing noises or voices talking when there is nobody around and nothing else to explain it?' (**auditory hallucinations**)
- 'How many voices are there?' (**type of auditory hallucination**)
- 'Do these voices speak directly to you or about you?' (**second or third person auditory hallucination respectively**)
- 'Do these voices ever make comments about what you're doing?' (**third person auditory hallucinations – running commentary**)
- 'Are you afraid that someone else is trying to harm you?' (**persecutory delusion**)
- 'Have you noticed that people are doing or saying things that have a special meaning to you?' 'When you watch television or read the newspaper do you ever worry that there are messages specifically for you?' (**delusions of reference**)
- 'Do you have any special powers or abilities?' (**grandiose delusions**)
- 'Have you ever felt that thoughts are being taken out of your mind?' (**thought withdrawal**)
- 'Have you ever experienced thoughts inside your head that are not yours and have been put there by someone else?' (**thought insertion**)
- 'Have you ever felt under the control of an outside force?' (**passivity phenomenon**)

MSE	**Appearance**	Can be normal (**positive**), or inappropriate with poor self-care (**negative**).
	Behaviour	Preoccupied, restless, noisy or suspicious (**positive**). A few show sudden, unexpected changes in behaviour. Withdrawn, poor eye contact and apathy (**negative**).
	Speech	May reflect underlying thought disorder (loosening of associations, pressured and distractible speech), interruptions to flow of thought (thought blocking), and poverty of speech (**negative**).
	Mood	Incongruity of affect or mood changes such as depression, anxiety or irritability. Flattened affect (**negative**).
	Thought	Delusions (e.g. persecutory, delusions of control, delusions of reference), thought insertion/withdrawal/broadcast, formal thought disorder (loosening of associations, word salad, concrete thinking, circumstantiality/tangentiality) (**all positive**).
	Perception	Hallucinations (especially third person auditory in nature) (**positive**).
	Cognition	Normal orientation. Attention and concentration often impaired (**positive**). May be evidence of premorbid cognitive impairment. Specific cognitive deficits (**negative**).
	Insight	Generally poor.

Ix
- **Blood tests: FBC** (anaemia, infection), **TFTs** (thyroid dysfunction can present with psychosis), **glucose** or **HbA1c** (as atypical antipsychotics can cause metabolic syndrome), **serum calcium** (hypercalcaemia can present with psychosis), **U&Es** and **LFTs** (assess renal and liver function before giving antipsychotics), **cholesterol** (as atypical antipsychotics cause metabolic syndrome), **vitamin B_{12} and folate** (deficiencies can cause psychosis).
- **Urine drug test: Illicit drugs** can cause and exacerbate psychosis.
- **ECG:** Antipsychotics cause **prolonged QT interval**.
- **CT scan:** To rule out organic causes such as **space-occupying lesions**.
- **EEG:** To rule out **temporal lobe epilepsy** as possible cause of **psychosis**.

DDx See *Fig. 4.1.1*, Overview of psychosis.

Management (includes NICE guidelines 2014)

- **Risk assessment** is vital and the use of the **Mental Health Act** may be required for those who refuse informal admission.
- The care of the schizophrenic patient is a joint effort between primary and secondary care and a combination of inpatient and outpatient care. Involvement of the psychiatric consultant, community psychiatric nurses, GPs, Crisis resolution team, social workers, carers and voluntary

organizations is essential. A **care programme approach** may be used (see *Chapter 1, Introduction to psychiatry*).

- For a first presentation of psychosis, the **early intervention in psychosis team** should be involved. They provide interventions targeted at reducing the duration of untreated psychosis (a strong prognostic indicator).

- It is essential to assess social circumstances and involve family where possible.

- The principle management of schizophrenia is outlined using the **bio-psychosocial model** (see *Table 4.2.2*).

Key facts 2: Poor prognostic factors for schizophrenia

Factors associated with poor prognosis:

- **Strong family history.**
- **Gradual onset.**
- **↓ IQ.**
- **Premorbid history of social withdrawal.**
- **No obvious precipitant.**

Table 4.2.2: Bio-psychosocial approach to the management of schizophrenia

Biological	
Antipsychotics (see *Fig. 4.2.2* and *Section 12.3*, Antipsychotics)	<ul><li>Antipsychotics can be broadly divided into **typical** and **atypical**.</li><li>**Atypical** antipsychotics are **first-line**, e.g. risperidone and olanzapine.</li><li>**Depot** formulations should be considered if the patient prefers or there is a problem with non-compliance.</li><li>**Clozapine** is the most effective antipsychotic and used for **treatment-resistant schizophrenia** (failure to respond to two other antipsychotics).</li></ul>
Adjuvants	<ul><li>**Benzodiazepines** can provide short-term relief of **behavioural disturbance**, insomnia, aggression and agitation.</li><li>**Antidepressants** and **lithium** can be used to **augment** antipsychotics.</li></ul>
ECT	<ul><li>May be appropriate in patients who are **resistant to pharmacological agents**. Effective for **catatonic schizophrenia**.</li></ul>
Psychological	
CBT	<ul><li>CBT is strongly recommended by NICE. **Reduces residual symptoms**.</li></ul>
Family intervention	<ul><li>Particularly useful for families of patients with schizophrenia who have persisting symptoms. **Psychoeducation** helps families **reduce high levels of expressed emotion** which reduces relapse rates.</li></ul>
Art therapy	<ul><li>NICE recommends art therapy (e.g. music, dancing, drama) for the alleviation of **negative symptoms** in young people.</li></ul>
Social skills training	<ul><li>Uses a **behavioural approach** to help patients improve **interpersonal**, **self-care** and **coping** skills needed in everyday life.</li></ul>

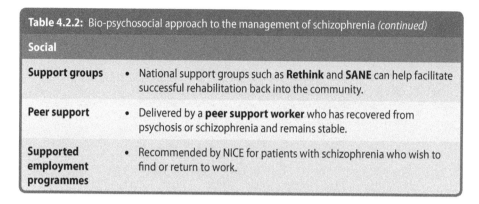

Table 4.2.2: Bio-psychosocial approach to the management of schizophrenia *(continued)*

Social	
Support groups	• National support groups such as **Rethink** and **SANE** can help facilitate successful rehabilitation back into the community.
Peer support	• Delivered by a **peer support worker** who has recovered from psychosis or schizophrenia and remains stable.
Supported employment programmes	• Recommended by NICE for patients with schizophrenia who wish to find or return to work.

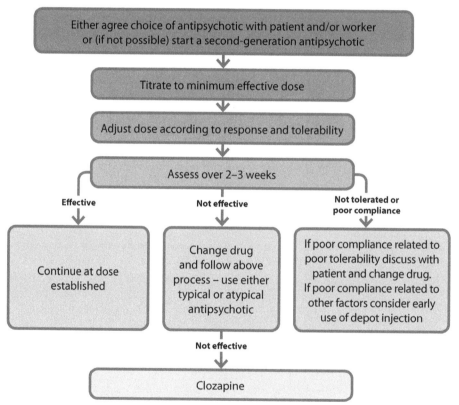

Fig. 4.2.2: Treatment of first-episode schizophrenia (adapted from *The Maudsley Prescribing Guidelines in Psychiatry*, 2015).

Self-assessment

A 22-year-old unmarried man presents to the clinic with his mother. He spends most of his time at home and refuses to go out at night alone. He states he saw lightning and is now convinced that the FBI is after him and that FBI agents gather information about his whereabouts. He believes that they are trying to control his thoughts and movement. He also hears them outside his house talking about how they will murder him. He appears suspicious, avoids eye contact, and his answers to questions are delayed, during which he appears internally preoccupied.

1. What is the most likely diagnosis? Name five differential diagnoses. *(3 marks)*
2. Which of Schneider's first rank symptoms is this patient suffering from? *(3 marks)*
3. What are the negative symptoms of schizophrenia? *(4 marks)*
4. What investigations would you perform on this patient and why? *(4 marks)*
5. Name an atypical antipsychotic that could be given to this patient. Name four side effects of this medication. *(5 marks)*
6. Name some potential psychosocial interventions for this patient. *(4 marks)*

Answers to self-assessment questions are to be found in *Appendix B*.

Chapter 5

Neurotic, stress-related and somatoform disorders

Definitions and epidemiology

- Neurosis is a collective term for psychiatric disorders **characterized by distress**, that are **non-organic**, have a **discrete onset** and where delusions and hallucinations are absent.

- **Anxiety** is an **unpleasant emotional state** involving **subjective fear** and **somatic symptoms**.

- Every human experiences anxiety, but if these anxieties become **excessive** or **inappropriate** they are described as an illness.

- The **Yerkes–Dodson law** states that anxiety can actually be beneficial up to a **plateau of optimal functioning**. Beyond this level of anxiety however, performance deteriorates (*Fig. 5.1.1*).

Fig. 5.1.1: Yerkes–Dodson curve.

- Anxiety disorders are **common** in primary and secondary care, with associated physical symptoms usually the cause of presentation, as opposed to psychological symptoms.

- The most common anxiety disorders, in order of **prevalence**, are **specific phobia, social phobia, generalized anxiety disorder, agoraphobia, panic disorder** and **OCD**.

- The one year **prevalence** of anxiety disorders is approximately **14%**.

ICD-10 Classification of neurotic and stress-related disorders

1. **Phobic anxiety disorders:** Agoraphobia (with or without panic disorder), social phobia, specific phobia.
2. **Other anxiety disorders:** Panic disorder, generalized anxiety disorder, mixed anxiety and depressive disorder.
3. **Obsessive–compulsive disorder:** Predominantly obsessional thoughts, predominantly compulsive thoughts, mixed.
4. **Reaction to severe stress and adjustment disorders:** Acute stress reaction, post-traumatic stress disorder, adjustment disorder.

Psychological
Anticipatory fear of impending doom, worrying thoughts, exaggerated startle response, restlessness, poor concentration and attention, irritability, depersonalization and derealization

Cardiovascular
Palpitations, chest pain

Respiratory
Hyperventilation, cough, chest tightness

Gastrointestinal
Abdominal pain ('butterflies'), loose stools, nausea and vomiting, dysphagia, dry mouth

Genitourinary
↑ Frequency of micturition, failure of erection, menstrual discomfort

Neuromuscular
Tremor, myalgia, headache, paraesthesia, tinnitus

Fig. 5.1.2: Common symptoms of neuroses.

Clinical features of neuroses

- **Common symptoms** that can feature in any anxiety disorder are shown in *Fig. 5.1.2.*
- Associated **cognitions** include **worries** or **fears** that are **inappropriate** or **excessive**.
- Associated **behaviours** include **avoidance** or **escape** from the situation that causes anxiety.
- **Depressive symptoms** are **very common** in patients with neuroses.
- In history taking the interviewer should ask about **rate of onset**, **duration** and **severity** of the anxiety, whether the anxiety arises **spontaneously** or in **response to a specific situation**, and whether there are any **psychiatric or medical conditions** which may predispose to anxiety.

Classification of neuroses

- Neuroses can be categorized based on the **nature** of the anxiety and the **circumstances** in which the anxiety occurs.
- Anxiety disorders can be divided into **two** main categories (*Fig. 5.1.3*):

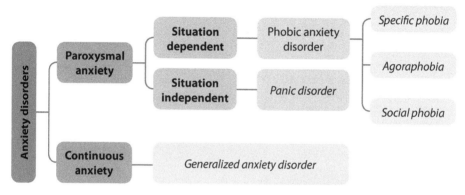

Fig. 5.1.3: The anxiety disorders.

1. **Generalized (free floating) anxiety: Present most of the time** and not associated with specific objects or situations. **Excessive or inappropriate worry** about **normal life events**. Typically **longer duration** (days, months or even years).
2. **Episodic (paroxysmal) anxiety:** Has an **abrupt onset** and occurs in **discrete episodes**. The episode of anxiety is **severe** with **strong autonomic symptoms**, but usually **short-lived** (typically less than one hour). Can occur in response to specific threats.

Conditions associated with anxiety

- There are many conditions associated with anxiety which can be divided into **medical**, **substance-related** and **psychiatric** (see *Table 5.1.1*).
- These are all potential **differential diagnoses** for a patient presenting with features of anxiety.

NOTE: Any **chronic condition** (e.g. COPD, CCF) may cause anxiety and depressive symptoms.

Table 5.1.1: Conditions associated with anxiety

Medical	Hyperthyroidism, hypoglycaemia, anaemia, phaeochromocytoma, Cushing's disease, chronic obstructive pulmonary disease (COPD), congestive cardiac failure (CCF), malignancies
Substance-related	• Intoxication: e.g. alcohol, cannabis, caffeine • Withdrawal: e.g. alcohol, benzodiazepine, caffeine • Side effects: e.g. thyroxine, steroids, adrenaline
Psychiatric	Eating disorders, somatoform disorders, depression, schizophrenia, OCD, post-traumatic stress disorder, adjustment disorder, anxious (avoidant) personality disorder

5.2 Generalized anxiety disorder

Generalized anxiety disorder (GAD) is a syndrome of **ongoing**, **uncontrollable**, **widespread worry** about many events or thoughts that the **patient recognizes** as **excessive** and **inappropriate**. Symptoms must be present on **most days** for at least **6 months** duration.

Pathophysiology/Aetiology

- The aetiology of GAD can be divided into **biological** and **environmental** causes (*Fig. 5.2.1*). Biological causes can further be split into **genetic** and **neurophysiological**.

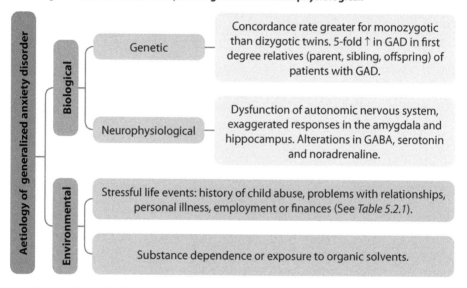

Aetiology of generalized anxiety disorder

Biological

- **Genetic** — Concordance rate greater for monozygotic than dizygotic twins. 5-fold ↑ in GAD in first degree relatives (parent, sibling, offspring) of patients with GAD.

- **Neurophysiological** — Dysfunction of autonomic nervous system, exaggerated responses in the amygdala and hippocampus. Alterations in GABA, serotonin and noradrenaline.

Environmental

- Stressful life events: history of child abuse, problems with relationships, personal illness, employment or finances (See *Table 5.2.1*).

- Substance dependence or exposure to organic solvents.

Fig. 5.2.1: Outline of the biological and environmental factors associated with GAD.

Epidemiology and risk factors (*Table 5.2.1*)

- GAD has a prevalence of **2–4%** in the general population.
- It is **more common in** ♀ at a ratio of **2:1**.

Table 5.2.1: Risk factors for GAD	
Predisposing	• Genetics, childhood upbringing, personality type and demands for high achievement. Being divorced. Living alone or as a single parent. Low socioeconomic status.
Precipitating	• Stressful life events such as domestic violence, unemployment, relationship problems and personal illness (e.g. chronic pain, arthritis, COPD).
Maintaining	• Continuing stressful events, marital status, living alone and ways of thinking which perpetuate anxiety (e.g. 'What will happen if others notice that I am anxious?').

Clinical features

- Clinical features of GAD can be divided into the areas shown in *Fig. 5.2.2*.
- **Common features** of presentation *specific* to GAD are listed below ('**WATCHERS**'):
  - **W**orry (excessive, uncontrollable)
  - **A**utonomic hyperactivity (sweating, ↑ pupil size, ↑ HR)
  - **T**ension in muscles/**T**remor
  - **C**oncentration difficulty/**C**hronic aches
  - **H**eadache/**H**yperventilation
  - **E**nergy loss
  - **R**estlessness
  - **S**tartled easily/**S**leep disturbance (difficulty getting to sleep then intermittent awakening and nightmares).

ICD-10 Criteria for GAD

A. A period of at least **6 months** with **prominent tension, worry** and **feelings of apprehension** about everyday events and problems.

B. At least **four** of the following symptoms with **at least one symptom of autonomic arousal**:
  - Symptoms of autonomic arousal: **palpitations, sweating, shaking/tremor, dry mouth**.
  - Other symptoms: See *Fig. 5.2.2*.

Diagnosis and investigations

Hx
- 'Talk me through a normal day in your life.' **(open question to identify anxiety)**
- 'Do you ever feel worried with your current state of affairs?', 'Do you worry excessively about minor things on most days of the week?', 'Would you say you are an anxious person?', 'Recently, have you been feeling anxious or on edge?' **(generalized worry)**
- 'Have you noticed any problems with your memory or concentration?' **(↓ concentration)**
- 'Do you ever lie awake at night worrying, or intermittently wake from sleep?', 'Do you ever have unpleasant dreams or nightmares?' **(sleep disturbance)**
- Ask about **somatic symptoms**, e.g. 'Do you ever feel the sensation of your heart beating abnormally fast or pounding on your chest?'

Symptoms concerning chest and abdomen

- Difficulty breathing
- Feeling of choking
- Chest pain or discomfort
- Nausea
- Abdominal distress or pain
- Loose motions.

Symptoms concerning the brain and mind

- Feeling dizzy or light headed
- Fear of dying
- Fear of losing control
- Derealization and depersonalization.

General symptoms

- Hot flushes or cold chills
- Numbness or tingling
- Headache.

Symptoms of tension

- Muscle tension, aches or pains
- Restlessness
- Feeling on edge
- Difficulty swallowing
- Sensation of lump in throat.

Non-specific symptoms

- Being startled
- Concentration difficulty and mind blanks
- Persistent irritability
- Sleep problems.

Fig. 5.2.2: Potential symptoms of GAD (*ICD-10*).

MSE		
Appearance and behaviour	Face looks worried with brow furrowed. Restless with tremor. Sweaty when you shake their hand. Hyperventilating. Lip biting. Pallor. Tense posture.
Speech	Trembling. Slow rate.
Mood	Anxious.
Thought	Repetitive worrying thoughts. Thoughts may concern personal health, safety of others or excessive worry about everyday events, e.g. relationships, finances.
Perception	No hallucinations.
Cognition	May complain of poor memory and reduced attention/concentration.
Insight	May or may not have insight.

NOTE: Observations may reveal a raised heart rate, respiratory rate and blood pressure.

Ix
- **Blood tests: FBC** (for infection/anaemia), **TFTs** (hyperthyroidism), **glucose** (hypoglycaemia).
- **ECG:** may show sinus tachycardia.
- **Questionnaires:** GAD-2, GAD-7, Beck's Anxiety Inventory, Hospital Anxiety and Depression Scale.

DDx
- **Other neurotic disorders:** panic disorder, specific phobias, OCD, PTSD.
- **Depression.**
- **Schizophrenia.**
- **Personality disorder** (e.g. anxious PD, dependent PD).
- **Excessive caffeine or alcohol consumption.**
- **Withdrawal from drugs.**
- **Organic:** anaemia, hyperthyroidism, phaeochromocytoma, hypoglycaemia (see *Table 5.1.1* in Introduction to anxiety disorders, for comprehensive list).

OSCE tips: Screening for other conditions

In an OSCE, it is very important to screen for depression and substance misuse in patients who you suspect have generalized anxiety disorder, as these conditions are strongly associated.

Management (includes NICE guidance 2011)

- The management of generalized anxiety disorder is based on the bio-psychosocial model:
  - Biological: The **first-line drug** treatment of choice is an **SSRI** (sertraline is recommended) which has anxiolytic effects. If this does not help an **SNRI** (e.g. venlafaxine or duloxetine) can be offered. If both of these are ineffective or not tolerated, **pregabalin** may be used. Medication should be continued for at least a year. **Benzodiazepines** should not be offered except as **short-term measures** during crises as they can cause dependence.

- Psychological: **Psychoeducational groups** are a *low intensity* form of psychological intervention. *High intensity* includes **cognitive behavioural therapy** and **applied relaxation** (practising techniques that lead to muscular or bodily relaxation, which can be applied in situations that trigger anxiety and worry).
- Social: Include **self-help methods** (such as writing down worrying thoughts and analysing them objectively) and **support groups**. **Exercise** should be encouraged and may benefit.
- **Co-morbid depression** or **substance misuse** should be treated (See *OSCE tips*).
- NICE suggests a **stepped care model** to determine the most effective interventions for patients with GAD (*Fig. 5.2.3*).

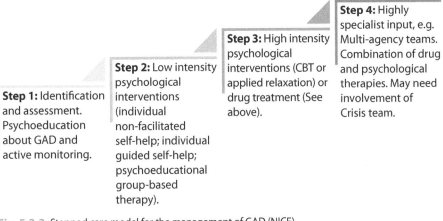

Step 1: Identification and assessment. Psychoeducation about GAD and active monitoring.

Step 2: Low intensity psychological interventions (individual non-facilitated self-help; individual guided self-help; psychoeducational group-based therapy).

Step 3: High intensity psychological interventions (CBT or applied relaxation) or drug treatment (See above).

Step 4: Highly specialist input, e.g. Multi-agency teams. Combination of drug and psychological therapies. May need involvement of Crisis team.

Fig. 5.2.3: Stepped care model for the management of GAD (NICE).

Self-assessment

A 35-year-old female presents to you complaining of longstanding tiredness. At first glance, she appears pale, worried and shaky. On questioning you discover she has been finding it difficult to get to sleep for the past year and when she does eventually get to sleep she is awoken by nightmares. Her mouth is constantly dry despite drinking plenty of water and she frequently gets chest tightness and feels sick. She is worried that this is all impacting on her job as a teacher. You suspect generalized anxiety disorder.

1. How long do symptoms need to be present for in order for this diagnosis to be made? *(1 mark)*
2. Give three investigations. *(3 marks)*
3. Other than dry mouth and chest pain, give six somatic symptoms of this disorder. *(3 marks)*
4. What is the first-line pharmacotherapy for this condition? *(1 mark)*
5. Give two psychosocial forms of management for this condition. *(2 marks)*

Answers to self-assessment questions are to be found in *Appendix B*.

Definition

- Phobia: is an **intense**, **irrational** fear of an **object**, **situation**, **place** or **person** that is recognized as **excessive** (out of proportion to the threat) or **unreasonable**.
- Agoraphobia: Agoraphobia literally means a 'fear of the marketplace'. It is a fear of **public spaces** or fear of entering a public space from which **immediate escape would be difficult** in the event of a panic attack.
- Social phobia **(social anxiety disorder):** A fear of **social situations** which may lead to **humiliation**, **criticism** or **embarrassment**.
- Specific (isolated) phobia: A fear restricted to a **specific object or situation** (excluding agoraphobia and social phobia).

Pathophysiology/Aetiology (*Table 5.3.1*)

Table 5.3.1: Aetiology of phobias	
Agoraphobia	Maintained by avoidance which prevents deconditioning and sets up a vicious cycle of anxiety.
Social phobia	Uncertain aetiology. Usually begins in late adolescence, an age at which people are concerned about the impression they make on others.
Specific phobia	Conditioning event in early life, i.e. a frightening experience. Possibly a role for learned behaviour, e.g. from parents (*Fig. 5.3.1*).

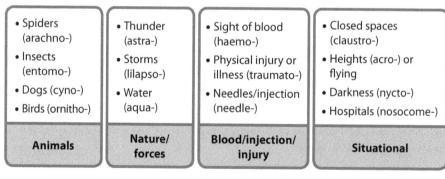

Animals	**Nature/ forces**	**Blood/injection/ injury**	**Situational**
• Spiders (arachno-) • Insects (entomo-) • Dogs (cyno-) • Birds (ornitho-)	• Thunder (astra-) • Storms (lilapso-) • Water (aqua-)	• Sight of blood (haemo-) • Physical injury or illness (traumato-) • Needles/injection (needle-)	• Closed spaces (claustro-) • Heights (acro-) or flying • Darkness (nycto-) • Hospitals (nosocome-)

Fig. 5.3.1: Some common specific phobias. Prefixes refer to the name of the phobia.

Epidemiology (Table 5.3.2) and risk factors (Table 5.3.3)

Table 5.3.2: Epidemiology of phobic anxiety disorders

Phobic anxiety disorder	1 year prevalence	Age of onset	♂:♀ ratio
Agoraphobia (affects up to 1/3 of those with panic disorder)	0.4%	Early adulthood (25–30 years of age)	2:1
Social phobia	1.2%	Usually adolescence	1:1
Specific phobia	3.5%	Usually childhood but can develop in later in life	1:1

Table 5.3.3: Risk factors for phobias

Aversive experiences (prior experiences with specific objects or situations)

Stress and negative life events

Other anxiety disorders

Mood disorders

Substance misuse disorders

Family history

Clinical features

- **Biological: Tachycardia** is the usual **autonomic response**, however in phobias of blood, injection and injury, a **vasovagal response** (bradycardia) is produced, commonly leading to fainting (**syncope**). For a complete list of biological symptoms see GAD, *Section 5.2*.
- **Psychological:** Include unpleasant **anticipatory anxiety**, **inability to relax**, urge to **avoid** the feared situation and, at extremes, a **fear of dying**.
- Agoraphobia is strongly linked to panic disorder. Indeed the *ICD-10* divides agoraphobia into: agoraphobia *with* panic disorder and agoraphobia *without* panic disorder.

ICD-10 Criteria		
Agoraphobia	**Social phobia**	**Specific phobia**
A. **Marked** and consistently manifest **fear in**, or **avoidance of**, at least **two** of the following: 1. Crowds 2. Public spaces 3. Travelling alone 4. Travelling away from home B. **Symptoms of anxiety** in the **feared situation** with at least **two symptoms** present together (and at least one symptom of autonomic arousal). See *Fig. 5.2.2* in GAD, *Section 5.2*.	A. **Marked fear** (*or* marked **avoidance**) of being the **focus of attention**, or fear of acting in a way that will be embarrassing or humiliating. B. At least **two symptoms** of anxiety in the feared situation plus one of the following: 1. **Blushing** 2. **Fear of vomiting** 3. **Urgency** or **fear of micturition/defecation**	A. **Marked fear** (*or* **avoidance**) of a **specific object or situation** that is not agoraphobia or social phobia. B. **Symptoms of anxiety** in the **feared situation**.

ICD-10 Criteria *(continued)*

Agoraphobia	Social phobia	Specific phobia
C. **Significant emotional distress** due to the avoidance, or anxiety symptoms. Recognized as **excessive** or **unreasonable**. D. **Symptoms restricted to** (or predominate in) **feared situation**.	C. **Significant emotional distress** due to the avoidance or anxiety symptoms. D. Recognized as **excessive** or **unreasonable**. E. **Symptoms restricted to** (or predominate in) **feared situation**.	C. **Significant emotional distress** due to the avoidance or anxiety symptoms. Recognized as **excessive** or **unreasonable**. D. **Symptoms restricted** to the **feared situation**.

Diagnosis and investigations

Hx
- 'What situations cause you anxiety or embarrassment?' **(specific phobia)**
- 'Do you get symptoms in situations from which escape would be difficult?', 'Do you get symptoms in places or situations where help may not be available?', 'Do you get symptoms while being in a crowd or travelling on public transport?' **(agoraphobia)**
- 'Do you ever worry about what people think of you? Does this worry ever lead to you avoiding certain situations?' **(social phobia)**
- 'Do you avoid any situation because you know you will feel panicky?' **(anticipatory anxiety)**

OSCE tips: Features that distinguish phobic anxiety disorders from GAD (**SS, AA, AA**)

Even if a patient is calm when you speak to them, you should screen for phobias as they are **restricting conditions** due to **avoidance of the feared stimulus**. **Three features** separate phobic anxiety from GAD.
1. Anxiety occurs in **S**pecific **S**ituations:
   - *Agoraphobia* – Public transport, supermarkets (especially waiting in queues), cinemas, empty streets.
   - *Social phobia* – Social gatherings, parties, public speaking, meetings, classrooms, eating in public.
2. There is **A**nticipatory **A**nxiety when there is a prospect of encountering the feared situation.
3. There is **A**ttempted **A**voidance of circumstances that precipitate anxiety.

MSE		
Appearance & Behaviour	Restless and wanting to escape. Pale, sweaty, hyperventilating. May lose consciousness (blood or injection phobia).	
Speech	May be trembling or they may become speechless.	
Mood	Anxious.	
Thought	Unpleasant feelings towards threat. Fear of situation. Desire to escape. Fear of dying.	
Insight	Poor when feared stimulus present. Good when separated from stimulus.	
NOTE: MSE will be largely normal unless exposed to the stimulus for phobia.		

Ix As symptoms occur in a defined situation, diagnosis is usually straightforward with minimal need for investigations. **Questionnaires** include the Social Phobia Inventory and Liebowitz Social Anxiety Scale.

DDx
- **Psychiatric:** Panic disorder, PTSD, anxious personality disorder, somatoform disorders, adjustment disorder, depression, schizophrenia (may avoid socializing because of paranoid delusions).
- **Organic:** See *Table 5.1.1* in *Section 5.1*, Overview of anxiety disorders.

Management (includes NICE guidance 2013)

General points
- Try to establish a **good rapport** with the patient. Remember, particularly with social phobia, it may have been very challenging for the patient to attend the appointment.
- Advise **avoidance of anxiety-inducing substances**, e.g. caffeine.
- Screen for significant co-morbidities such as **substance misuse** and **personality disorders**.
- **Refer to a specialist** if there is a risk of **self-harm**, **suicide**, **self-neglect** or **significant co-morbidity**.

Management of the three phobic anxiety disorders (Table 5.3.4)

Table 5.3.4: Management of agoraphobia, social phobia and specific phobia	
Agoraphobia	• **CBT** is the psychological intervention of choice. The behavioural component includes graduated exposure and desensitization. **Graduated exposure** techniques such as walking increased distances from home day by day, can be used. • **SSRIs** are the first-line pharmacological agent.
Social phobia	• **CBT** (individual or group) specifically designed for social phobia. **Graduated exposure** to feared situations is included both within treatment sessions and as homework. • **Pharmacological interventions** include **SSRIs** (escitalopram or sertraline), **SNRIs** (venlafaxine) or if no response to these, a **MAOI** (moclobemide). • **Psychodynamic psychotherapy** for those who decline CBT or medication.
Specific phobia	• The mainstay of treatment is **exposure** either using self-help methods or more formally through **CBT**. • **Benzodiazepines** may be used as anxiolytics in the short term (due to risk of dependence) for instance if a patient needs an urgent CT scan and they are claustrophobic.

Self-assessment

A 35-year-old man experiences intense worry a few weeks before scheduled airline travel. However, he is required to fly several times every year with his work. He developed this 3 years ago following an extremely turbulent flight. He has recurring, vivid images of himself dying in a blazing crash while flying. He is hyperaware of any sound and unexpected movements of the plane. Over the last few months, he has been drinking excessive amounts of alcohol in an attempt to control his symptoms.

1. What type of phobia does this man have? *(1 mark)*
2. Give common examples of other types of this phobia. *(2 marks)*
3. What are the two other types of phobia and how would you differentiate between them? *(3 marks)*
4. How could this patient be managed? *(3 marks)*
5. What three features separate phobic anxiety disorders from GAD? *(3 marks)*

Answers to self-assessment questions are to be found in *Appendix B*.

Panic disorder is characterized by **recurrent**, **episodic**, **severe** panic attacks, which are **unpredictable** and **not restricted** to any particular situation or circumstance.

Pathophysiology/Aetiology (Table 5.4.1)

Table 5.4.1: Aetiology of panic disorder	
Biological	**Genetics:** Along with OCD, it is one of the most heritable anxiety disorders. **Neurochemical:** Post synaptic hypersensitivity to serotonin and adrenaline. **Sympathetic nervous system** (SNS): Fear or worry stimulates the SNS → ↑cardiac output which can lead to further anxiety.
Cognitive	Misinterpretation of somatic symptoms (e.g. fear that palpitations will lead to a heart attack).
Environmental	Presence of life stressors can lead to panic disorder.

Epidemiology and risk factors (Table 5.4.2)

- Panic disorder has a prevalence of **1%** in the general population.
- It is **three times** more common in ♀.
- The usual age of onset is **late adolescence**.

Table 5.4.2: Risk factors for panic disorder		
Family history	Major life events	Age (20–30)
Recent trauma	Females	Other mental disorders
White ethnicity	Asthma	Cigarette smoking
Medication (e.g. benzodiazepine withdrawal)		

Clinical features (see ICD-10 criteria)

- Panic symptoms usually **peak within 10 minutes** and **rarely persist beyond an hour**.

ICD-10 Criteria for the diagnosis of panic disorder

A. **Recurrent panic attacks** that are **not consistently associated with a specific situation or object**, and often occur **spontaneously**. The panic attacks are not associated with marked exertion or with exposure to dangerous or life-threatening situations.

B. Characterized by ALL of the following: (1) **Discrete episode** of **intense fear** or **discomfort**; (2) **Starts abruptly**; (3) Reaches a **crescendo within a few minutes** and **lasts at least some minutes**; (4) At least one symptom of **autonomic arousal**: palpitations, sweating, shaking/tremor, dry mouth; (5) **Other symptoms:** See GAD, *Section 5.2*.

OSCE tips: A useful mnemonic for some of the key features of panic disorder is 'PANICS Disorder'

Palpitations, **A**bdominal distress, **N**umbness/Nausea, **I**ntense fear of death, **C**hoking feeling/ **C**hest pain, **S**weating/**S**haking/**S**hortness of breath, **D**epersonalization/**D**erealization.

Diagnosis and investigations

Hx
- 'Are you generally anxious or are there periods where you are anxiety-free?' **(episodic)**
- 'Can you predict when these attacks will come on?' **(unpredictable)**
- 'Have you ever been so frightened that you felt your heart was pounding and that you might die?' **(intense fear and anxiety)**
- 'Are you worried about your health or any other specific things?' **(major life stressors)**

MSE The MSE findings in panic disorder (if the patient is having a panic attack when seen, which may not be the case) will be largely the same as in GAD (see *Section 5.2*). However, features of **appearance and behaviour** may be more intense such as hyperventilation and restlessness.

Ix As for generalized anxiety disorder (see *Section 5.2*).

DDx
- **Psychiatric:** Other anxiety disorders (e.g. generalized anxiety disorder, phobic anxiety disorder), dissociative disorder, bipolar affective disorder, depression, schizophrenia, adjustment disorder.
- **Organic:** Phaeochromocytoma, hyperthyroidism, hypoglycaemia, carcinoid syndrome, arrhythmias, alcohol/substance withdrawal (see *Table 5.1.1* in Overview of anxiety disorders).

Key facts 1: Comparing GAD, panic disorder and phobic anxiety

	GAD	Panic disorder	Phobic anxiety
Age of onset	*Variable:* adolescence to late adulthood	Late adolescence to early adulthood	Childhood to late adolescence
When does it occur?	Persistent	Episodic	Situational
Associated behaviour	Agitation	Escape	Avoidance
Cognition	Constant worry	Fear of symptoms	Fear of situation
Associations	Depression	Depression, agoraphobia, substance misuse	Substance misuse

Management (includes NICE guidance 2011)

- **SSRIs** are **first-line** but if they are not suitable, or there is no improvement after **12 weeks**, then a **TCA**, e.g. **imipramine** or **clomipramine** may be considered. *Benzodiazepines should not be prescribed.*
- **CBT** is the psychological intervention of choice, focusing on recognition of panic triggers.
- **Self-help methods** include **bibliotherapy** (giving written information on panic disorder and how to overcome it), **support groups** and **encouraging exercise** to promote good health.
- **NICE** offers a **stepped care approach** (*Fig. 2.4.1*).

Step 1: Recognition and diagnosis	**Step 2:** Treatment in primary care	**Step 3:** Review and consideration of alternative treatments	**Step 4:** Review and referral to specialist mental health services	**Step 5:** Care in specialist mental health services
Making the diagnosis and identifying common co-morbidities such as depression and substance misuse.	Includes recommendations for psychological therapies, medications and self-help strategies.	Describes reassessment and consideration of alternative treatments if initial therapy has failed.	States that if two interventions have been offered and there is no improvement in symptoms then referral should be made to specialists.	Discusses reassessment in secondary care, of the patient's social circumstances and environment, and advises shared decisions to be made.

Fig. 5.4.1: Stepped care model for management of panic disorder.

Self-assessment

A 38-year-old man presents to A&E for the second time in 3 weeks with sudden onset shortness of breath, chest pain, palpitations, dizziness, and sweating. He tells the doctor he is afraid of having a heart attack and fears he is going to die whenever it happens. He has stopped driving and has started avoiding crowded areas for fear of inducing further attacks. His past medical history is unremarkable. Cardiac investigations, including ECG and troponin, during both admissions were normal.

1. What is this man describing? *(1 mark)*
2. Name three organic disorders that may present similarly. *(3 marks)*
3. What are the differences between GAD, panic disorder and phobic anxiety disorders? *(3 marks)*
4. What is the first-line management for this condition? *(1 mark)*

Answers to self-assessment questions are to be found in *Appendix B*.

Definitions

There are several conditions associated with reactions to stressful events:

- **Post-traumatic stress disorder (PTSD):** Is an **intense**, **prolonged**, **delayed** reaction following exposure to an **exceptionally traumatic event**. This chapter will focus on PTSD.
- **Abnormal bereavement:** Normal bereavement goes through a number of stages in response to loss of a loved one. Abnormal bereavement has a **delayed onset**, is **more intense** and **prolonged** (**>6 months**). The impact of their loss overwhelms the individual's coping capacity.
- **Acute stress reaction:** An abnormal reaction to **sudden stressful events** (see *Key facts*).
- **Adjustment disorder:** Normal adjustment refers to psychological reactions involved in adapting to new circumstances. Adjustment disorder is when there is **significant distress** (greater than expected), accompanied by an **impairment in social functioning** (see *Key facts*).

Pathophysiology/Aetiology

- The most important component of aetiology is an **exceptionally stressful event** in which the individual was **involved directly** or as a **witness** (see *Table 5.5.1*).
- Not all individuals who experience the same traumatic experience go on to develop PTSD, thus suggesting a pre-existing **vulnerability**. Twin studies of Vietnam War veterans suggest that part of the vulnerability may be **genetic** (see *Table 5.5.2*).
- **Cognitive theories** suggest that failure to process emotionally charged events causes memories to persist in an unprocessed form which can intrude into conscious awareness.

Epidemiology and risk factors

- Approximately **3%** of adults in England suffer from PTSD.
- **25–30%** of individuals experiencing a traumatic event may go on to develop PTSD.
- It can affect people of all ages, but is **more common in** ♀ (♀:♂ ratio is **2:1**).

Table 5.5.1: Traumatic events

Severe assault (e.g. physical or sexual abuse, robbery, mugging).
Major natural disaster (e.g. earthquakes, floods).
Serious road traffic accident.
Observer/survivor of civilian disaster (e.g. acts of terrorism, the Holocaust).
Involvement in wars (e.g. World War II, Vietnam War).
Freak occurrences (e.g. near drowning when on holiday).
Physical torture.
Prisoner of war or **hostage situation**.
Hearing about **unexpected injury** or **violent death** of a **family member** or **friend**.

Table 5.5.2: Risk factors for PTSD

Exposure to a major traumatic event	• Professions at risk (armed forces, police, fire services, journalists, doctors), groups at risk (refugees, asylum seekers).
Pre-trauma	• Previous trauma, history of mental illness, females, low socio-economic background, childhood abuse.
Peri-trauma	• Severity of trauma, perceived threat to life, adverse emotional reaction during or immediately after event.
Post-trauma	• Concurrent life stressors, absence of social support.

Clinical features

PTSD symptoms must occur **within 6 months** of the event and can be divided into **four** categories:

1. **Reliving** the situation (persistent, intrusive, involuntary): Flashbacks, vivid memories, nightmares, distress when exposed to similar circumstances as the stressor.

2. **Avoidance:** Avoiding reminders of trauma (e.g. associated people or locations), excessive rumination about the trauma, inability to recall aspects of the trauma.

3. **Hyperarousal:** Irritability or outbursts, difficulty with concentration, difficulty with sleep, hypervigilance, exaggerated startle response.

4. **Emotional numbing:** Negative thoughts about oneself, difficulty experiencing emotions, feeling of detachment from others, giving up previously enjoyed activities.

ICD-10 Criteria for the diagnosis of PTSD

A. **Exposure to a stressful event** or situation of extremely threatening or catastrophic nature (would likely cause distress in almost anyone).

B. **Persistent remembering** ('reliving') of the stressful situation.

C. Actual or preferred **avoidance of similar situations** resembling or associated with the stressor.

D. Either (1) or (2)

   1. **Inability to recall** some important aspects of the period of exposure to the stressor.

   2. Persistent symptoms of **increased psychological sensitivity** and **arousal**.

E. Criteria B, C & D all occur **within 6 months** of the stressful event, or the end of a period of stress.

Diagnosis and investigations

Hx
- 'Has there been any traumatic incident or event in your life recently which may account for how you are feeling?' **(exposure to stressful event)**
- 'Do you ever get any flashbacks, vivid memories or nightmares about the events that took place?' **(reliving the situation)**
- 'Do you find yourself constantly thinking about the same thing?' **(rumination)**
- 'Have you had any problems with sleep since the event?', 'Are you feeling more irritable or having trouble concentrating?', 'Do you get startled easily?' **(hyperarousal)**

OSCE tips: Normal bereavement reaction (*Fig. 5.5.1*)

In an OSCE, you may have a patient with severe symptoms after the loss of a loved one. Remember whilst it may be tempting to diagnose PTSD, **bereavement is a unique traumatic stress** which is a **normal human experience**. Bereavement reactions are natural and not coded for in *ICD-10*. Normal bereavement should not extend over **6 months**; if it does, **abnormal bereavement** or **adjustment disorder** should be considered.

MSE	**Appearance & Behaviour**	Hypervigilance ('on edge'), exaggerated startle reaction, may have features of anxiety or depression, e.g. poor eye contact.
	Speech	Slow rate. Trembling. Non-spontaneous.
	Mood	Anxious.
	Thought	Pessimistic. Reliving or remembering of the event.
	Perception	No hallucinations. May have illusions.
	Cognition	Poor attention and concentration.
	Insight	Good.

Ix
- **Questionnaires:** Trauma Screening Questionnaire (TSQ), Post-traumatic diagnostic scale.
- **CT head:** if head injury suspected.

DDx
- **Psychiatric:** Adjustment disorder, acute stress reaction, bereavement, dissociative disorder, mood or anxiety disorders, personality disorder.
- **Organic:** Head injury (result of traumatic event), alcohol/substance misuse.

Stages of Grief
'DABDA'

DENIAL:
Temporary denial of reality as emotionally overwhelmed

↓

ANGER:
Intense emotions expressed as anger

↓

BARGAINING:
Negotiating a compromise in order to reduce grief

↓

DEPRESSION:
Depressed mood

↓

ACCEPTANCE:
Acceptance and reorganization of life

Fig. 5.5.1: Kübler–Ross stages of grief.

Management (includes NICE guidance)

Key facts 1: Acute stress reaction and adjustment disorder (*ICD-10*)

Acute stress reaction
Exposure to an **exceptional physical or mental stressor** (e.g. physical assault, road traffic accident) followed by an **immediate onset** of symptoms (**within one hour**). Divided into **mild**, **moderate** or **severe** based on extent of symptoms. Possible symptoms include **anxiety symptoms** (see *Section 5.2*, GAD), **narrowing of attention**, **apparent disorientation**, **anger** or **verbal aggression**, **despair** or **hopelessness**, **uncontrollable** or **excessive grief**. Symptoms must begin to diminish within **8 hours** (for *transient* stressors) or **48 hours** (for *continued* stressors).

Adjustment disorder
Identifiable (**non-catastrophic**) **psychosocial stressor** (e.g. redundancy, divorce) **within one month** of onset of symptoms. Symptoms are variable but can be of the types found in the affective disorders or the neurotic disorders (but not severe enough to be classed as a specific psychiatric disorder). The symptoms must be present for **less than 6 months**.

PTSD where symptoms are present within 3 months of a trauma

- **Watchful waiting** may be used for mild symptoms lasting <4 weeks.
- Military personnel have access to treatment provided by the armed forces.
- **Trauma-focused CBT** should be given at least once a week for 8–12 sessions.
- **Short-term drug treatment** may be considered in the acute phase for management of **sleep disturbance** (e.g. zopiclone).
- **Risk assessment** is important to assess risk for neglect or suicide.

PTSD where symptoms have been present >3 months after a trauma

- All sufferers should be offered a course of **trauma-focused psychological intervention**.
- The two options for psychological intervention are **CBT** and **eye movement desensitization and reprocessing (EMDR)**. The goal of **EMDR** is to reduce distress in the shortest period of time. It is a form of psychotherapy, with one technique involving eye movements to help the brain process traumatic events (see *Section 12.1*, Psychotherapies).
- **Drug treatment** should be considered when: (1) **little benefit** from **psychological therapy**; (2) **patient preference** not to engage in psychological therapy; (3) **co-morbid depression** or **severe hyperarousal** which would benefit from psychological interventions.
- **Paroxetine**, **mirtazapine**, **amitriptyline** and **phenelzine** are licensed for treatment of PTSD in the UK. Evidence for paroxetine is weaker than the other three drugs. Practically, amitriptyline and phenelzine are rarely used as a result of their side effects and tolerability.

Self-assessment

A 35-year-old lady presents to you with her husband. She does not speak much English and it transpires that she has recently arrived in the country (3 months ago) from Syria to be with her husband. The husband describes that she has been increasingly detached since she has been in the country and has given up activities that she previously enjoyed. She is easily startled, for instance when the cat makes a noise. On further questioning you discover that in her last few days in Syria, she saw her close friend being brutally assaulted to the point of hospitalization. You suspect PTSD.

1. Name six symptoms of PTSD. *(3 marks)*
2. Within how many months of the traumatic event do symptoms have to occur? *(1 mark)*
3. Name two distinguishing features between PTSD and adjustment disorder. *(2 marks)*
4. Name two non-pharmacological management strategies for PTSD. *(2 marks)*
5. Give two examples of antidepressants which are commonly used to treat PTSD. *(2 marks)*

Answers to self-assessment questions are to be found in *Appendix B*.

Definition

Obsessive–compulsive disorder (OCD) is characterized by **recurrent obsessional thoughts** or **compulsive acts**, or commonly both. It is ranked by the WHO as one of the top ten most disabling illnesses in terms of impact upon quality of life.

Obsessions: **Unwanted intrusive thoughts**, **images** or **urges** that **repeatedly** enter the individual's mind. They are **distressing** for the individual who attempts to **resist** them and recognizes them as absurd (**egodystonic**) and a product of their **own mind**.

Compulsions: **Repetitive**, **stereotyped behaviours** or **mental acts** that a person feels **driven** into performing. They are **overt** (observable by others) or **covert** (mental acts not observable).

Pathophysiology/Aetiology

There are a number of theories for the aetiology of OCD:

- Biological: Related to ↓ **serotonin** and abnormalities of the frontal cortex and basal ganglia. Twin and family studies suggest a **genetic contribution** to OCD particularly with paediatric onset. **Childhood group A beta-haemolytic streptococcal infection** may have a role in causing OCD symptoms by setting up an autoimmune reaction which damages the basal ganglia (this is called PANDAS).

- Psychoanalytic: Filling the mind with obsessional thoughts in order to prevent undesirable ideas from entering consciousness.

- Behavioural: Compulsive behaviour is learned and maintained by **operant conditioning**. The anxiety created by the obsession is reduced by performing the compulsion, and subsequently the need to perform the compulsion is increased.

OCD has strong associations with other psychiatric disorders: **depression (30%)**, **schizophrenia (3%)**, **Sydenham's chorea**, **Tourette's syndrome** and **anorexia nervosa**.

Epidemiology and risk factors

- The prevalence of OCD ranges from **0.8–3%**.
- It is **most common in early adulthood** and is **equally common in ♂ and ♀**.
- OCD is **more common** in the **relatives of OCD patients** than it is in the general population.
- **Carrying out the compulsive act** (e.g. washing) is likely to exacerbate the obsession and is thus a maintaining factor.
- **Developmental factors** such as neglect, abuse, bullying and social isolation may have a role.

ICD-10 Criteria for the diagnosis of OCD

A. Either obsessions or compulsions (or both) present on **most days** for a period of **at least 2 weeks**.

B. Obsessions (thoughts, ideas or images) or compulsions (acts) share a number of features (see *Clinical features*), ALL of which must be present.

C. The obsessions or compulsions cause **distress** or **interfere** with the subject's **social** or **individual** functioning, usually by wasting time.

NOTE: The diagnosis can be specified as 'predominantly obsessional thoughts or ruminations', 'predominantly compulsive acts', or 'mixed obsessional thoughts and acts'.

Clinical features

- Common obsessions and compulsions are illustrated in *Fig. 5.6.1*. The most common *obsession* is that of being **contaminated (38%)** and the most common *compulsion* is **checking (29%)** followed closely by **washing/cleaning (27%)**.

Obsessions	Compulsions
• Contamination (e.g. from dirt, viruses, germs, bodily fluids) • Fear of harm (e.g. door locks not safe) • Excessive concern with order or symmetry • Others: sex, violence, blasphemy, doubt	• Checking e.g. gas taps, water taps, doors (O) • Cleaning, washing (O) • Repeating acts e.g. counting (C), arranging objects (O) • Mental compulsions e.g. special words repeated in a set manner (C) • Hoarding (O)

Fig. 5.6.1: Obsessions and compulsions (C = covert; O = overt).

- Obsessions or compulsions must share **ALL** of the following features (**FORD Car**):

1. **Failure to resist:** At least one obsession or compulsion is present which is unsuccessfully resisted.
2. **Originate** from patient's mind: Acknowledged that the obsessions or compulsions originate from their own mind, and are not imposed by outside persons or influences.
3. **Repetitive and Distressing:** At least one obsession or compulsion must be present which is acknowledged by the patient as excessive or unreasonable.
4. **Carrying out the obsessive thought** (or compulsive act) is **not in itself pleasurable**, but reduces anxiety levels.

- Obsessions create **anxiety** which continues to build until a compulsion is carried out in order to provide **relief**. This vicious cycle is known as the **OCD cycle** (*Fig. 5.6.2*).

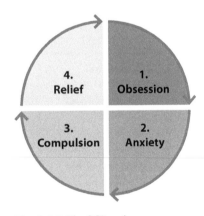

Fig. 5.6.2: The OCD cycle.

Diagnosis and investigations

Hx
- 'Do you have any distressing thoughts that enter your mind despite trying hard to resist them?', 'Is there any unwanted thought that keeps bothering you that you would like to get rid of but cannot?' **(obsessions)**
- 'Do you worry about contamination with dirt even after washing?', 'Do you repeatedly check things you have already done?', 'Do you find yourself having to touch, count and arrange things many times?', 'Do you wash or clean a lot? Do you check things a lot?', 'Are you concerned about putting things in a specific order, or do you get upset by not completing tasks?' **(compulsions)**
- 'Do your daily activities take a long time to finish?' **(due to carrying out compulsions)**

MSE
- Patient may be on edge (easily startled). May look visibly worried or lost in thought. May be constantly checking doors or fidgety with hands (as they can't wash them).
- May demonstrate increasing levels of **anxiety** if unable to succumb to compulsion (*Fig. 5.6.2*).
- **Thoughts** are **unwanted**, **intrusive** and **uncomfortable** for the patient.
- Obsessions can be distracting and lead to **poor concentration**.
- **Insight** is usually very **good** (as they recognize the thoughts are a product of their own mind).

OSCE tips 1: Exploring risk and co-existing psychiatric conditions

After exploring the patient's main obsessive–compulsive features, it is important to assess the impact of the obsessions and compulsions on the person's life and to assess risk, because these often are very distressing for the patient. Patients commonly have co-existing depression, anxiety disorders, substance misuse, eating disorders and body dysmorphic disorder, and therefore these should also be assessed for.

Ix **Questionnaires:** Yale–Brown obsessive–compulsive scale (Y-BOCS) → 10-item questionnaire with each item graded from 0–4; e.g. Time occupied by obsessive thoughts (0 = none, 4 = extreme, >8 hours/day).

DDx

Obsessions *and* compulsions	Primarily obsessions	Primarily compulsions	Organic
• **Eating disorders** (AN and BN) • **Anankastic personality disorder** • **Body dysmorphic disorder:** Preoccupation with an imagined defect in physical appearance, resulting in time-consuming behaviours, e.g. mirror gazing	• **Anxiety disorders** (e.g. phobic anxiety) • **Depressive disorder** • **Hypochondriacal disorder** • **Schizophrenia**	• **Tourette's syndrome** • **Kleptomania** (inability to refrain from stealing items)	• **Dementia** • **Epilepsy** • **Head injury**

Management (includes NICE guidance)

There are two main strategies to the treatment of OCD:

1. CBT (including ERP – exposure and response prevention)

- **ERP** is a technique in which patients are repeatedly exposed to the situation which causes them anxiety (e.g. exposure to dirt) and are prevented from performing the repetitive actions which lessen that anxiety (e.g. washing their hands). After initial anxiety on exposure, the levels of anxiety gradually decrease.

2. Pharmacological therapy

- **SSRIs** are the drug of choice in OCD. NICE recommends **fluoxetine, fluvoxamine, paroxetine, sertraline** or **citalopram**.
- **Clomipramine** is an alternative drug therapy. This can be combined with citalopram in more severe cases. Alternatively, an **antipsychotic** can be added in with an SSRI or clomipramine.

General points

- **Psychoeducation, distracting techniques** and **self-help books** can be used.
- Any potential **suicide risk** should be identified and managed.
- **Co-morbid depression** should be identified and treated.
- Method of treatment depends upon the **degree of functional impairment** (*Fig. 5.6.3*). This ranges from **mild** (limited impact on ADL) to **severe** (obsessional slowness that greatly impacts performance).

Low intensity psychological intervention (defined as <10 hours of therapist input per patient)
Mild

SSRI or high intensity psychological intervention
Moderate

Combined SSRI and CBT (with ERP)
Severe

Fig. 5.6.3: Management of OCD based on severity of functional impairment.

Self-assessment

A 22-year-old male student presents with his girlfriend who is worried about him as he spends at least 4 hours in the bathroom every day. He reluctantly describes a 6-month history of recurrent thoughts that he has specks of blood on his hands and feet. He has to shower exactly 12 times a day to be cleansed of this blood. He realizes that this is abnormal.

1. What is the most likely diagnosis? *(1 mark)*
2. Provide two differential diagnoses. *(2 marks)*
3. What further questions may you want to ask in order to confirm the diagnosis? *(2 marks)*
4. What is the main difference in thought process here compared to in schizophrenia? *(1 mark)*
5. What group of pharmacological agents would you give to this patient? Give an example of a drug belonging to this category that is commonly used. *(2 marks)*
6. What psychotherapy would you suggest for this patient and what sub-type? *(2 marks)*

Answers to self-assessment questions are to be found in *Appendix B*.

Somatoform disorders are a group of disorders whose symptoms are suggestive of, or take the form of, a **physical disorder** but in the **absence of a physiological illness**, leading to the presumption that they are caused by **psychological factors**. Sufferers **repeatedly seek medical attention** even when it has consistently failed to benefit them.

Dissociative (conversion) disorders are characterized by symptoms which cannot be explained by a medical disorder and where there are **convincing associations in time** between **symptoms and stressful events**, problems or needs. The unpleasant stressful events or problems are 'converted' into the symptoms.

Pathophysiology/Aetiology

- The cause of **somatoform disorders** is **multifactorial** (see *Table 5.7.1*). Patients adopt the **sick role**, which provides relief from stressful or unachievable interpersonal expectations (**primary gain**). This offers attention, care from others and sometimes even financial rewards (**secondary gain**) in many societies.

Table 5.7.1: Pathophysiology of somatoform disorders	
Biological	• Possible implication of neuroendocrine genes. Studies indicate a genetic component.
Psychological	• A high proportion of those with PTSD suffer from somatoform disorders. • Association between somatization and physical or sexual abuse.
Social	• Adopting of the 'sick role' in order to gain relief from stress.

- **Dissociative disorders** *must* be causally linked in time with stressful life events, problems or needs.

- As the name suggests, dissociative (conversion) disorders require **two** processes to occur:

  1. **Dissociation:** A process of 'separating off' certain memories from normal consciousness. This is a **psychological defence mechanism** that is used to cope with emotional conflict that is so distressing for the patient, that it is prevented from entering their conscious mind.

  2. **Conversion:** Distressing events are transformed into physical symptoms. This, like somatoform disorders, can lead to **primary** and **secondary gain** (*Fig. 5.7.1*).

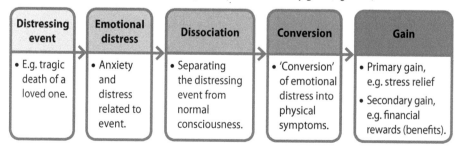

Distressing event	Emotional distress	Dissociation	Conversion	Gain
• E.g. tragic death of a loved one.	• Anxiety and distress related to event.	• Separating the distressing event from normal consciousness.	• 'Conversion' of emotional distress into physical symptoms.	• Primary gain, e.g. stress relief • Secondary gain, e.g. financial rewards (benefits).

Fig. 5.7.1: Sequence of events in dissociative (conversion) disorders.

Epidemiology and risk factors (*Table 5.7.2*)

- The prevalence of somatoform disorders in the UK is **0.1–2%**.
- They are **more common in** ♀ than in ♂ and are likely to begin **before the age of 30**.
- Prevalence of dissociative disorder in clinical settings in Western societies is between **2 and 6 per 100** for ♀.

Table 5.7.2: Risk factors for somatoform and dissociative disorders ('   ')

Childhood abuse
Reinforcement of illness behaviours
Anxiety disorders
Mood disorders
Personality disorders
Social stressors

Clinical features

- **Dissociative (conversion) disorder** is named on the premise that painful or stressful thoughts are subconsciously 'converted' into more bearable physical symptoms by the patient.
- There are different types of dissociative disorder based on the feature which predominates, and these are summarized in *Fig. 5.7.2*.
- The different types of **somatoform disorder** (based on *ICD-10*) are illustrated in *Fig. 5.7.3*.

Dissociative amnesia	• Amnesia, either partial or complete for recent events or problems that were traumatic or stressful. Too extensive and persistent to be explained by ordinary forgetfulness.
Dissociative fugue	• An unexpected physical journey away from usual surroundings followed by amnesia for the journey. Self-care is maintained.
Dissociative stupor	• Profound reduction in, or absence of, voluntary movements, speech and normal responses to stimuli. Normal muscle tone.
Trance and possession disorders	• **Trance:** temporary alteration in state of consciousness. • **Possession:** absolute conviction by the patient that they have been taken over by a spirit, power or person.
Dissociative motor disorders	• Loss of the ability to perform movements that are under voluntary control (including speech) or ataxia.
Dissociative convulsions	• Sudden, unexpected spasmodic movements that resemble epilepsy but without loss of consciousness.
Dissociative anaesthesia and sensory loss	• Partial or complete loss of cutaneous sensation, vision, hearing or smell.

Fig. 5.7.2: *ICD-10* categories of dissociative (conversion) disorder.

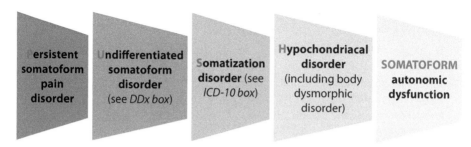

Fig. 5.7.3: *ICD-10* categories of somatoform disorders [Mnemonic] 'PUSHY SOMATOFORM patients' (on the basis that somatoform disorder patients **push** for investigations to be performed).

Somatization disorder

- Also known as **Briquet's syndrome**.
- **Multiple, recurrent** and **frequently changing** physical symptoms **not explained by a physical illness**.
- More common in ♀ (♀:♂ ratio is **10:1**).
- Common symptoms are listed in *Fig. 5.7.4*.
- **Long history of contact** with **medical services**.
- Often dependent on analgesics with a degree of functional impairment.

ICD-10 Criteria for somatization disorder

Somatization disorder requires all **four** to be present:

A. At least **2 years' duration** of **physical symptoms** that **cannot be explained** by any **detectable physical disorder**.

B. **Preoccupation** with symptoms causes **physical distress** which leads to them **seeking repeated medical consultations** and **requesting investigations**.

C. **Continuous refusal** by patients to **accept reassurance** from doctors that there is no physical cause for their symptoms.

D. A total of **six** or more symptoms (*Fig. 5.7.4*).

Gastrointestinal	Cardiovascular	Genitourinary	Others
• Abdominal pain • Nausea and vomiting • Bloating • Regurgitation • Loose bowel motions • Swallowing difficulty	• Chest pain • Breathlessness at rest • Palpitations	• Dysuria • Frequency • Incontinence • Vaginal discharge • Menstrual problems	• Discolouration or itching of skin • Arthralgia • Paraesthesia in limbs • Headaches • Visual disturbance

Fig. 5.7.4: Common symptoms in somatization disorder.

Hypochondriacal disorder

- Patient **misinterprets normal bodily sensations**, which leads them to the **non-delusional preoccupation** that they have a **serious physical disease**, e.g. cancer.

- They **refuse to accept reassurances** from doctors.

- **Dysmorphophobia** (body dysmorphic disorder) is a variant where there is an **excessive preoccupation** with **barely noticeable or imagined defects** in their **physical appearance** (e.g. the size and shape of their nose). The preoccupation causes significant distress (*Fig. 5.7.5*).

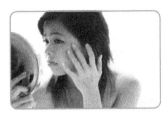

Fig. 5.7.5: An illustration of dysmorphophobia.

Somatoform autonomic dysfunction

- Symptoms are related to the **autonomic nervous system**.

- Symptoms of autonomic arousal are attributed by patients to a physical disorder of **one or more** of the **cardiovascular, respiratory, upper GI, lower GI** or **genitourinary systems**.

- **Multiple autonomic symptoms** must be present such as **palpitations, tremor, sweating, dry mouth, flushing** and **hyperventilation**. Symptoms may be **objective** (sweating, tremor) or **subjective** (pain, paraesthesia).

- Patients attribute symptoms to a specific system under autonomic control. For instance respiratory (**psychogenic hyperventilation**), gastrointestinal (**irritable bowel syndrome**) or cardiovascular (**Da Costa's syndrome**).

Persistent somatoform pain disorder

- **Persistent** (of at least **6 months'** duration) and **severe pain** that cannot be fully explained by a physical disorder.

- Pain usually occurs as a result of **psychosocial stressors** and **emotional difficulties**.

- Differs from somatization disorder in that **pain is the primary feature** and multiple symptoms from different systems are **not** present.

Diagnosis and investigations

Hx
- 'Do you ever worry about your health?'
- 'Do you feel that you have multiple medical problems?'
- 'Are you worried about having a potentially serious medical condition?'
- 'Do you get frustrated when doctors tell you that you are fit and well?'
- 'Have there been any stressful events in your life that may have triggered your symptoms?'

MSE
MSE findings in the areas of **appearance, behaviour** and **mood** may reflect underlying mood or anxiety disorders. **Thoughts** will show preoccupation with physical symptoms and overvalued ideas of having a serious medical condition. **Insight** into having a *psychiatric* illness will likely be clouded.

Ix **NOTE:** Somatoform disorders are often a **diagnosis of exclusion**. However, certain features point in the direction of a somatoform disorder. These include: (1) Multiple symptoms, often occurring in different organ systems; (2) Vague symptoms that exceed objective findings; (3) Chronic course; (4) Presence of a mental health disorder; (5) History of extensive diagnostic testing; and (6) Rejection of previous physicians.

- A **thorough physical examination** and **investigations** are performed to rule out an organic cause depending on the symptoms present.
- **Blood tests: FBC** (anaemia, infection), **U&Es** (electrolyte disturbance), **LFTs** (liver or biliary pathology), **CRP** (infection, inflammation), **TFTs** (thyroid dysfunction).
- **Further investigations:**
  A. Gastrointestinal symptoms: AXR, stool culture, OGD, colonoscopy, diagnostic laparoscopy.
  B. Cardiovascular symptoms: ECG, 24 hr tape, ECHO, angiogram.
  C. Genitourinary symptoms: urine dipstick, MSU, cystoscopy.

DDx
- **Somatoform disorders:** Somatization disorder, hypochondriacal disorder, somatoform autonomic dysfunction, persistent somatoform pain disorder, undifferentiated somatoform disorder (**less severe variation on somatization disorder** with a duration of at least **6 months – commonest** somatoform disorder).
- **Dissociative (conversion) disorder.**
- **Factitious disorder.**
- **Malingering.**
- **Other psychiatric disorders:** Mood disorder, psychotic disorder, anxiety disorder, PD.
- **Multi-systemic disease**, e.g. connective tissue disorders and inflammatory bowel disease.

Key facts 1: Malingering and factitious disorder

- In both malingering and factitious disorder (also known as Munchausen's syndrome) **physical or psychological symptoms are intentionally** produced, i.e. faked. The difference between the two is the patient's **motive** behind mimicking the symptoms (*Fig. 5.7.6*).
- **Malingering:** Patient **seeks advantageous consequences** of being diagnosed with a medical condition. For instance, evading criminal prosecution or receiving government benefits (i.e. **secondary gain**).
- **Factitious disorder (Munchausen's syndrome):** The individual wishes to **adopt the 'sick role'** in order to receive the care of a patient, for **internal emotional gain** (i.e. **primary gain**).

Factitious disorder	Malingering	Somatoform disorder	Dissociative disorder
'I want to go to the hospital to be looked after.'	'If I go to the hospital, I may receive compensation.'	'I think I have a serious illness and need to go to hospital for more tests!'	'Ever since I lost my job, I've been feeling so unwell!'

Fig. 5.7.6: Comparison between factitious disorder, malingering, somatoform disorders and dissociative disorder.

Management (Fig. 5.7.7)

Biological therapies

For somatoform and dissociative disorders include **antidepressants** (primarily SSRIs) for any **underlying mood disorder**. **Physical exercise** enhances self-esteem and can be particularly helpful in **dysmorphophobia**.

Psychological therapies

The **mainstay** of management is **cognitive behavioural therapy** usually in short courses. Developing certain coping strategies can also be very useful.

Social therapies

From a **social** perspective, **stress-relieving activities** such as meditation and long walks can prove effective, as well as interventions reducing specific causes of stress (e.g. marriage counselling). It may be appropriate to interview/**involve family** members who serve to reinforce the sick role.

Biological
- Antidepressants
- Physical exercise

Psychological
- CBT
- Coping strategies

Social
- Encourage pleasurable private time
- Involve family where appropriate

Fig. 5.7.7: Bio-psychosocial management of medically unexplained symptoms.

OSCE tips: Explaining the diagnosis to a patient with a somatoform disorder

- A major obstacle in the management of patients with somatoform disorder or indeed any functional symptoms is that they often feel that doctors don't believe them and they feel that this brings into question their integrity. Therefore, good communication is of the utmost importance.
- **Discuss investigations** → 'The results of my examination and of the tests we conducted show that you do not have a life-threatening illness. However, what you are describing is something that I see often, but it is not completely understood.'

OSCE tips: Explaining the diagnosis to a patient with a somatoform disorder *(continued)*

- **Brief explanation** → 'Many people like yourself have physical symptoms that we cannot find a reason for. We usually call these 'medically unexplained symptoms' or 'functional illness'.
- **Placing a positive spin** → 'I would like to reassure you however, that there are still ways we can help you. We can help train your body to work normally again but may be unable to pinpoint the exact cause.'
- **Relate to a disorder they are more familiar with** → 'We know that most physical illnesses get worse if the patient feels tense or down, for example stress makes asthma worse, and therefore I feel that if we manage other problems in your life you will automatically feel better within yourself. How do you feel about this?'

NOTE: Allow the patient to query what you have said. Allow carers and relatives to be involved in the consultation.

Consultation for patient with medically unexplained symptoms

DO:	DO NOT:
• Focus on symptoms and their effect on the patient. • Match your explanation using their own words. • Share your uncertainty; discuss possible test results and their implications. • Reach a shared understanding; listen to their ideas, concerns and expectations. • Acknowledge the importance of the patient's views and circumstances. • Agree to follow-up arrangements.	• Focus exclusively on a diagnosis or give a diagnosis when there is uncertainty. • Dismiss the symptoms as normal without matching your explanation to the patient's concerns. • Treat symptoms with medications anyway. • Assume what the patient wants. • Judge the patient or be critical of their behaviours. • Ignore or dismiss psychological cues. • Enforce psychosocial explanations, as this can lead to defensiveness.

Self-assessment

A 22-year-old female university student sought medical attention for recurrent physical symptoms which consisted of gastrointestinal difficulties, dysmenorrhoea, nausea, weakness, malaise, fatigue, headaches, back pain, and insomnia. Her mother took her to numerous physicians in an attempt to find solutions to her complaints. As a result, she has had many investigations performed for which no biological cause has been identified. Both she and her mother refuse to accept reassurance that there is no physical cause for her symptoms.

1. List four differential diagnoses. *(2 marks)*
2. What type of somatoform disorder is this lady likely to be suffering from and why? *(2 marks)*
3. Name the three other types of somatoform disorders. *(3 marks)*
4. What is the difference between a somatoform disorder and malingering or factitious disorder? *(3 marks)*

Answers to self-assessment questions are to be found in *Appendix B.*

Chapter 6

Eating disorders

Anorexia nervosa (AN) is an **eating disorder** characterized by **deliberate weight loss**, an **intense fear of fatness**, **distorted body image**, and **endocrine disturbances**.

The aetiology of AN is generally considered to be **multifactorial**, and can be divided into predisposing, precipitating and perpetuating factors (see *Table 6.1.1*).

Table 6.1.1: Aetiological factors in AN			
	Biological	**Psychological**	**Social**
Predisposing	• Genetics: Monozygotic twin studies have higher concordance rates than dizygotic twins. • Family history: First degree relatives have higher incidence of eating disorders. • Female. • Early menarche.	• Sexual abuse. • Preoccupation with slimness. • Dieting behaviours starting in adolescence. • Low self-esteem. • Premorbid anxiety or depressive disorder. • Perfectionism, obsessional/anankastic personality.	• Western society: Pressure to diet in a society that emphasizes that being thin is beauty. • Bullying at school revolving around weight. • Stressful life events.
Precipitating	• Adolescence and puberty.	• Criticism regarding eating, body shape or weight.	• Occupational or recreational pressure to be slim, e.g. ballet dancers, models.
Perpetuating (maintaining)	• Starvation leads to neuroendocrine changes that perpetuate anorexia.	• Perfectionism, obsessional/anankastic personality.	• Occupation. • Western society.

- AN affects ♀ more than ♂ (**10:1**).
- Estimated incidence is **0.4 per 1000 yearly in** ♂ and approximately **9 in 1000** ♀ will experience it at some point in their lives.
- The typical **age of onset** is **mid-adolescence**.

Clinical features

- The defining clinical features of AN are described in the *ICD-10* box.

> **ICD-10 Criteria for the diagnosis of AN: 'FEED'**
>
> - **Fear of weight gain**.
> - **Endocrine disturbance** resulting in **amenorrhoea** in females and loss of sexual interest and potency in males.
> - **Emaciated** (abnormally low body weight): >15% below expected weight or BMI <17.5 kg/m².
> - **Deliberate weight loss** with ↓ food intake or ↑ exercise.
> - **Distorted body image** (*Fig. 6.1.1*).
>
> **NOTE:** The above features must be present for at least **3 months** and there must be the **ABSENCE** of (1) **recurrent episodes of binge eating**; (2) **preoccupation with eating/craving to eat**.

- Other features include **PP**, **SS**:

  - **Physical:** Fatigue, hypothermia, bradycardia, arrhythmias, peripheral oedema (due to hypoalbuminaemia), headaches, lanugo hair (*Fig. 6.1.2*).

  - **Preoccupation with food:** Dieting, preparing elaborate meals for others.

  - **S**ocially isolated, **S**exuality feared.

  - **S**ymptoms of depression and obsessions.

> **Key facts 1:** Working out BMI
>
> **Body mass index = weight (kg) ÷ [height (m)]²**
>
> BMI <18.5 kg/m² = **underweight**
> BMI 18.5–24.9 kg/m² = **normal**
> BMI 25–29.9 kg/m² = **overweight**
> BMI ≥30 kg/m² = **obese**

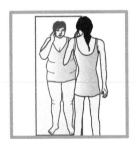

Fig. 6.1.1: Distorted body image.

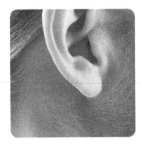

Fig. 6.1.2: Lanugo hair.

> **OSCE tips:** Anorexia nervosa vs. bulimia nervosa
>
> | Anorexia nervosa | Bulimia nervosa |
> | --- | --- |
> | <ul><li>Are significantly underweight.</li><li>Are more likely to have endocrine abnormalities such as amenorrhoea.</li><li>Do not have strong cravings for food.</li><li>Do not binge eat.</li><li>May have compensatory weight loss behaviours (excluding purging).</li></ul> | <ul><li>Are usually normal weight/overweight.</li><li>Are less likely to have endocrine abnormalities.</li><li>Have strong cravings for food.</li><li>Have recurrent episodes of binge eating.</li><li>Have compensatory weight loss behaviours.</li></ul> |

Diagnosis and investigations

Hx
- 'Some people find body shape and weight to be very important to their identity. Do you ever find yourself feeling concerned about your weight?' **(fear of weight gain)**
- 'What would be your ideal target weight?' **(overvalued ideas about weight)**
- 'The obvious methods people use to lose weight are to eat less and exercise more. Are these things that you personally do?' **(deliberate weight loss)**
- 'When women lose significant weight, their periods have a tendency to stop. Has this happened in your case?' **(amenorrhoea)**
- Also ask *specifically* about **physical symptoms** of anorexia nervosa e.g. fatigue and headaches.

MSE

Appearance & Behaviour	Thin, weak, slow, anxious. May try to disguise emaciation with makeup. Baggy clothes. Dry skin. Lanugo hair.
Speech	May be slow, slurred, or normal.
Mood	Can be low with co-morbid depression, or euthymic.
Thought	Preoccupation with food, overvalued ideas about weight and appearance.
Perception	No hallucinations.
Cognition	Either normal or poor if physically unwell with complications.
Insight	Often poor.

NOTE: A full systems examination should be carried out to find out the degree of emaciation, to exclude differential diagnoses and to look for possible complications (see *Key facts 2*).

Ix
- **Blood tests: FBC** (anaemia, thrombocytopenia, leukopenia), **U&Es** (↑ urea and creatinine if dehydrated, ↓ potassium, phosphate, magnesium and chloride), **TFTs** (↓T_3 and T_4), **LFTs** (↓ albumin), **lipids** (↑ cholesterol), **cortisol** (↑), **sex hormones** (↓ LH, FSH, oestrogens and progestogens), **glucose** (↓), **amylase** (pancreatitis is a complication).
- **Venous blood gas (VBG):** Metabolic alkalosis (vomiting), metabolic acidosis (laxatives).
- **DEXA scan:** To rule out osteoporosis (if suspected).
- **ECG:** Arrhythmias such as sinus bradycardia and prolonged QT are associated with AN patients.
- **Questionnaires:** e.g. eating attitudes test (EAT).

DDx
- **Bulimia nervosa.**
- **Eating disorder not otherwise specified (EDNOS):** see *Key facts 3*.
- **Depression.**
- **Obsessive–compulsive disorder.**
- **Schizophrenia:** Delusions about food.
- **Organic causes of low weight:** Diabetes, hyperthyroidism, malignancy.
- **Alcohol** or **substance misuse**.

Key facts 2: Complications of AN

Metabolic	Hypokalaemia, hypercholesterolaemia, hypoglycaemia, impaired glucose tolerance, deranged LFTs, ↑ urea and creatinine (if dehydrated), ↓ potassium, ↓ phosphate, ↓ magnesium, ↓ albumin and ↓ chloride.
Endocrine	↑ Cortisol, ↑ growth hormone, ↓ T_3 and T_4, ↓ LH, FSH, oestrogens and progestogens leading to amenorrhoea. ↓ Testosterone in men.
Gastrointestinal	Enlarged salivary glands, pancreatitis, constipation, peptic ulcers, hepatitis.
Cardiovascular	Cardiac failure, ECG abnormalities, arrhythmias, ↓ BP, bradycardia, peripheral oedema.
Renal	Renal failure, renal stones.
Neurological	Seizures, peripheral neuropathy, autonomic dysfunction.
Haematological	Iron deficiency anaemia, thrombocytopenia, leucopenia.
Musculoskeletal	Proximal myopathy, osteoporosis.
Others	Hypothermia, dry skin, brittle nails, lanugo hair, infections, suicide.

Key facts 3: Other eating disorders

Bulimia nervosa	Recurrent episodes of binge eating and compensatory behaviour (any one or a combination of vomiting, fasting, or excessive exercise) in order to prevent weight gain (see *Section 6.2*, Bulimia nervosa).
Binge eating disorder	Recurrent episodes of binge eating without compensatory behaviour such as vomiting, fasting, or excessive exercise.
EDNOS or atypical eating disorder	One third of patients referred for eating disorders have EDNOS (eating disorders not otherwise specified). EDNOS closely resembles anorexia nervosa, bulimia nervosa, and/or binge eating, but does not meet the precise diagnostic criteria.

Management (includes NICE guidance)

- The management of AN is outlined using the **bio-psychosocial model** (*Fig. 6.1.3*).
- **Risk assessment** for suicide and medical complications is absolutely vital.
- **Psychological treatments** should normally be for at least **6 months' duration**.
- The aim of treatment as an **inpatient** is for a weight gain of **0.5–1 kg/week** and as an **outpatient** of **0.5 kg/week**.
- Patients are at risk of **refeeding syndrome** which causes metabolic disturbances (e.g. ↓ phosphate) and other complications (see *Key facts 4*).
- **Hospitalization** is necessary for **medical** (severe anorexia with BMI <14 or severe electrolyte abnormalities) and **psychiatric** (suicidal ideation) reasons.
- In cases where insight is clouded, use of the **MHA** (or **Children Act**) for life-saving treatment, may be required.

Biological
• **Treatment of medical complications**, e.g. electrolyte disturbance
• **SSRI**s for co-morbid depression or OCD

Psychological
• **Psycho-education** about nutrition
• **Cognitive behavioural therapy**
• **Cognitive analytic therapy**
• **Interpersonal psychotherapy**
• **Family therapy**

Social
• **Voluntary organizations**
• **Self-help groups**

Fig. 6.1.3: Bio-psychosocial approach to AN.

Key facts 4: Refeeding syndrome

- A potentially life-threatening syndrome that results from food intake (whether parenteral or enteral) after **prolonged starvation** or **malnourishment**, due to changes in **phosphate**, **magnesium** and **potassium**.
- It occurs as a result of an **insulin surge** following increased food intake.
- Biochemical features include fluid balance abnormalities, **hypokalaemia**, **hypomagnesaemia**, **hypophosphataemia** and **abnormal glucose metabolism**.
- The phosphate depletion causes reduction in cardiac muscle activity which can lead to **cardiac failure**.
- Prevention: Measure serum electrolytes prior to feeding and **monitor refeeding bloods daily**, start at 1200 kcal/day and gradually increase every 5 days, monitor for signs such as **tachycardia** and **oedema**.
- If electrolyte levels are low, they will need to be replaced either orally or intravenously depending upon the severity of electrolyte depletion.

Self-assessment

A 16-year-old girl, accompanied by her mother, presents to her GP complaining of fatigue for 6 months. The doctor observes the patient is rather petite and is wearing an oversized, baggy dress. No signs are found on examination. During the examination the patient mentions how fat she has become. She weighs 42 kg and measures 160 cm. Her mother is concerned as her daughter has been eating only one small meal a day and exercising excessively, and seems uninterested in her friends. Her periods have also stopped.

1. Work out the girl's BMI. *(2 marks)*
2. What is the most likely diagnosis? Name two differential diagnoses. *(2 marks)*
3. What are the defining features of this condition? *(4 marks)*
4. Give four complications of this condition? *(4 marks)*
5. Outline the management strategy for this patient. *(4 marks)*

Answers to self-assessment questions are to be found in *Appendix B*.

Bulimia nervosa (BN) is an **eating disorder** characterized by **repeated episodes** of **uncontrolled binge eating** followed by **compensatory weight loss behaviours** and **overvalued ideas** regarding 'ideal body shape/weight'.

Pathophysiology/Aetiology

- The aetiology of BN is very similar to AN, but whereas there is a clear genetic component in AN, the **role of genetics in BN is unclear**.
- When patients with BN binge due to **strong cravings**, they tend to feel guilty and as a result undergo **compensatory behaviours** such as **vomiting**, using **laxatives**, **exercising excessively** and **alternating with periods of starvation**. This may result in large fluctuations in weight, which reinforce the compensatory weight loss behaviour, setting up a vicious cycle (*Fig. 6.2.1*).

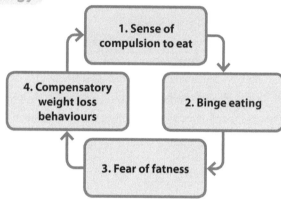

Fig. 6.2.1: The vicious cycle of BN.

Epidemiology and risk factors (Table 6.2.1)

- BN typically occurs in **young women**. The estimated prevalence in women aged **15–40** is **1–2%**.
- Whereas AN is thought to be more prevalent in higher socioeconomic classes, **BN has equal socioeconomic class distribution**.

Table 6.2.1: Risk factors for bulimia nervosa

	Biological	Psychological	Social
Predisposing	• Female sex • Family history of eating disorder, mood disorder, substance misuse or alcohol abuse • Early onset of puberty • Type 1 diabetes • Childhood obesity	• Physical or sexual abuse as a child • Childhood bullying • Parental obesity • Pre-morbid mental health disorder • Preoccupation with slimness • Parents with high expectations • Low self-esteem	• Living in a developed country • Profession (e.g. actors, dancers, models, athletes) • Difficulty resolving conflicts

Table 6.2.1: Risk factors for bulimia nervosa *(continued)*

	Biological	Psychological	Social
Precipitating	• Early onset of puberty/ menarche	• Perceived pressure to be thin may come from culture (e.g. Western society, media and profession) • Criticism regarding body weight or shape	• Environmental stressors • Family dieting
Perpetuating	• Co-morbid mental health problems	• Low self-esteem, perfectionism • Obsessional personality	• Environmental stressors

OSCE tips 1: BN and other co-morbid psychiatric conditions

BN commonly co-exists with the following psychiatric disorders and it is hence important to screen for them:
1. Depression
2. Anxiety
3. Deliberate self-harm
4. Substance misuse
5. Emotionally unstable (borderline) personality disorder.

Clinical features

ICD-10 Criteria for the diagnosis of BN: 'Bulimia Patients Fear Obesity'	
1. **B**ehaviours to prevent weight gain (compensatory)	Compensatory weight loss behaviours include: **self-induced vomiting**, alternating periods of **starvation**, **drugs** (laxatives, diuretics, appetite suppressants, amphetamines, and thyroxine), and **excessive exercise**. **NOTE:** diabetics may omit or reduce insulin dose.
2. **P**reoccupation with eating	A **sense of compulsion** (craving) to eat which leads to bingeing. There is typically regret or shame after an episode.
3. **F**ear of fatness	Including a **self-perception** of being too fat.
4. **O**vereating	At least **two episodes per week** over a period of **3 months**.

Other features include:
- **Normal weight:** Usually the potential for weight gain from bingeing is counteracted by the weight loss/purging behaviours.
- **Depression and low self-esteem.**
- **Irregular periods.**

- **Signs of dehydration:** ↓ blood pressure, dry mucous membranes, ↑ capillary refill time, ↓ skin turgor, sunken eyes.
- **Consequences of repeated vomiting and hypokalaemia** (see *Key facts 2* and 3).

Key facts 1: Subtypes of bulimia nervosa

There are **two** subtypes of BN:
1. **Purging type:** The patient uses self-induced vomiting and other ways of expelling food from the body, e.g. use of laxatives, diuretics and enemas.
2. **Non-purging type:** Much less common. Patients use excessive exercise or fasting after a binge. Purging-type bulimics may also exercise and fast but this is not the main form of weight control for them.

NOTE: ICD-10 does not differentiate between purging and non-purging.

OSCE tips 2: Anorexia vs. bulimia

Amenorrhoea	**B**inge eating
No friends (socially isolated)	**U**se of drugs to prevent weight gain
Obvious weight loss	**L**ow potassium
Restriction of food intake	**I**rregular periods
Emaciated	**M**ood disturbances
Xerostomia (dry mouth)	**I**rrational fear of fatness
Irrational fear of fatness	**A**lternating periods of starvation
Abnormal hair growth (lanugo hair)	

Key facts 2: Hypokalaemia (↓ K⁺)

- A potentially life-threatening complication of excessive vomiting.
- Low potassium (<3.5 mmol/L) can result in muscle weakness, cardiac arrhythmias and renal damage.
- Mild hypokalaemia requires oral replacement with potassium-rich foods (e.g. bananas) and/or oral supplements (Sando-K).
- Severe hypokalaemia requires hospitalization and intravenous potassium replacement.

Diagnosis and investigations

 Hx
- 'Do you ever feel that your eating is getting out of control?' **(binge eating)**
- 'After an episode of eating what you later feel is too much, do you ever make yourself sick so that you feel better?' **(compensatory self-induced vomiting)**
- 'Have you ever used medication to help control your weight?' **(self-induced purging)**
- 'Do you ever feel a strong craving to eat?' **(preoccupation with food)**
- 'Do you ever get muscle aches?', 'Do you ever have the sensation that your heart is beating abnormally fast?' **(complications of hypokalaemia)**
- Ask specifically about complications of repeated vomiting (see *Key facts 3*).
- Screen for other co-morbid psychiatric conditions (see *OSCE tips 1*).

MSE		
	Appearance & Behaviour	May have appearance and behaviour consistent with depression or anxiety. Likely normal weight. Parotid swelling. Russell's sign (*Fig. 6.2.2*). Sunken eyes (dehydration).
	Speech	Slow or normal.
	Mood	Low.
	Thought	Preoccupation with body size and shape. Preoccupation with eating. Guilt.
	Perception	Normal.
	Cognition	Either normal or poor.
	Insight	Usually has good insight.

Ix

- **Blood tests:** FBC, U&Es, amylase, lipids, glucose, TFTs, magnesium, calcium, phosphate.
- **Venous blood gas:** May show metabolic alkalosis.
- **ECG:** Arrhythmias as a consequence of hypokalaemia (ventricular arrhythmias are life threatening), classic ECG changes (prolongation of the PR interval, flattened or inverted T waves, prominent U waves after T wave).

DDx

- **Anorexia nervosa** – with bulimic symptoms.
- **EDNOS** (**E**ating **D**isorder **N**ot **O**therwise **S**pecified).
- **Kleine–Levin syndrome:** Sleep disorder in adolescent males characterized by recurrent episodes of binge eating and hypersomnia.
- **Depression.**
- **Obsessive–compulsive disorder.**
- **Organic causes of vomiting**, e.g. gastric outlet obstruction.

Key facts 3: Physical complications of repeated vomiting	
Cardiovascular	Arrhythmias, mitral valve prolapse, peripheral oedema.
Gastrointestinal	Mallory–Weiss tears, ↑ size of salivary glands especially parotid (*Fig. 6.2.2*).
Metabolic/Renal	Dehydration, hypokalaemia, renal stones, renal failure.
Dental	Permanent erosion of dental enamel secondary to vomiting of gastric acid (*Fig. 6.2.2*).
Endocrine	Amenorrhoea, irregular menses, hypoglycaemia, osteopenia.
Dermatological	Russell's sign (calluses on back of hand due to abrasion against teeth).
Pulmonary	Aspiration pneumonitis.
Neurological	Cognitive impairment, peripheral neuropathy, seizures.

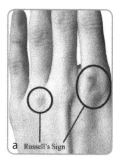
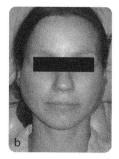
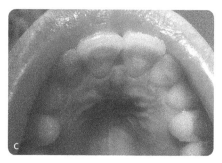

Fig. 6.2.2: Complications of repeated vomiting. (a) **Russell's sign**; (b) **Bilateral parotid swelling**; and (c) **Dental erosion**.

Management

- The management of BN is based on the bio-psychosocial model:
    - Biological: A trial of antidepressant should be offered and can ↓ frequency of binge eating/ purging. **Fluoxetine** (usually at high dose, 60 mg) is the SSRI of choice. Treat medical complications of repeated vomiting, e.g. potassium replacement. Treat co-morbid conditions (see *OSCE tips 1*).
    - Psychological: **Psychoeducation** about nutrition, CBT for bulimia nervosa (**CBT-BN** is a specifically adapted form of CBT). **Interpersonal psychotherapy** is an alternative.
    - Social: **Food diary** to monitor eating/purging patterns, **techniques to avoid bingeing** (eating in company, distractions), **small, regular meals, self-help programmes**.
- From a biological perspective, **electrolytes should be monitored carefully** for any potential disturbances, and should be replaced accordingly where appropriate.
- **Risk assessment** for suicide. Co-morbid depression and substance misuse are common.
- **Inpatient treatment** is required for cases of **suicide risk** and **severe electrolyte imbalances**.
- The **Mental Health Act** is not usually required, as BN patients have **good insight** and are motivated to change.
- Approximately **50%** of BN patients make a **complete recovery** in comparison with AN where roughly 20% make a full recovery.

Self-assessment

A 25-year-old female vegetarian presents to you very distressed. She describes a 3-year history of strong cravings for food, resulting in sessions of binge eating. To make herself feel better she states that she deliberately vomits five times a day and compulsively exercises for 2 hours a day.

1. Which eating disorder is the most likely diagnosis? Name two differentials. *(3 marks)*
2. What are the four diagnostic features of this condition based on ICD-10? *(4 marks)*
3. What is the most important complication of repeated vomiting? How would you test for this in a laboratory? *(2 marks)*
4. Give two further complications for repeated episodes of vomiting. *(2 marks)*
5. Outline the management of this condition in the community. *(3 marks)*

Answers to self-assessment questions are to be found in *Appendix B*.

Chapter 7

Alcohol and substance misuse

7.1 Substance misuse

The **ICD-10** classifies substance misuse disorders according to the **type of substance** (see *Table 7.1.1*) and the **type of disorder** (see *ICD-10 box*).

ICD-10 Criteria for substance misuse

1. **Acute intoxication:** The acute, usually transient, effect of the substance.
2. **Harmful use:** Recurrent misuse associated with physical, psychological and social consequences, but without dependence.
3. **Dependence syndrome** (see *Key facts 1*): Prolonged, compulsive substance use leading to addiction, tolerance and the potential for withdrawal syndromes.
4. **Withdrawal state:** Physical and/or psychological effects from complete (or partial) cessation of a substance after prolonged, repeated or high level of use.
5. **Psychotic disorder:** Onset of psychotic symptoms *within 2 weeks* of substance use. Must persist for *more than 48 hours*.
6. **Amnesic syndrome:** Memory impairment in recent memory (impaired learning of new material) and ability to recall past experiences. Also defect in recall, clouding of consciousness and global intellectual decline.
7. **Residual disorder:** Specific features (flashbacks, personality disorder, affective disorder, dementia, persisting cognitive impairment) *subsequent* to substance misuse.

Pathophysiology/Aetiology (*Fig. 7.1.1*)

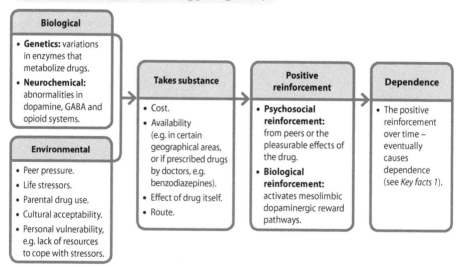

Fig. 7.1.1: Factors involved in, and chain of events leading to, substance dependence.

Table 7.1.1: Drug misuse

Group	Examples	Route PO: oral IV: intravenous IN: intranasal	Effects (psychological)	Effects (physical)	Withdrawal state (if applicable) At least 3 signs needed
Opiates	Morphine, diamorphine (heroin), codeine, methadone	Morphine (PO, IV), diamorphine (IN, IV, smoked), codeine/ methadone (PO)	Apathy, disinhibition, psychomotor retardation, impaired judgement and attention, drowsiness, slurred speech	Respiratory depression, hypoxia, ↓ BP, hypothermia, coma, pupillary constriction	Craving, rhinorrhoea, lacrimation, myalgia, abdominal cramps, N+V, diarrhoea, pupillary dilatation, piloerection, ↑ HR/↑ BP
Cannabinoids	Cannabis	PO, smoked	Euphoria, disinhibition, agitation, paranoid ideation, temporal slowing (time passes slowly), impaired judgement/ attention/reaction time, illusions, hallucinations	Increased appetite, dry mouth, conjunctival injection, ↑ HR	Anxiety, irritability, tremor of outstretched hands, sweating, myalgia
Sedative-hypnotics	Benzodiazepines, barbiturates	PO, IV	Euphoria, disinhibition, apathy, aggression, anterograde amnesia, labile mood	Unsteady gait, difficulty standing, slurred speech, nystagmus, erythematous skin lesions, ↓ BP, hypothermia, depression of gag reflex, coma	Tremor of hands, tongue or eyelids, N+V, ↑ HR, postural ↓ BP, headache, agitation, malaise, transient illusions/ hallucinations, paranoid ideation, grand mal convulsions

Table 7.1.1: Drug misuse *(continued)*

Group	Examples	Route PO: oral IV: intravenous IN: intranasal	Effects (psychological)	Effects (physical)	Withdrawal state (if applicable) At least 3 signs needed
Stimulants	Cocaine, crack cocaine, ecstasy (MDMA), amphetamine	Cocaine, crack cocaine (IN, IV, smoked), ecstasy (PO), amphetamine (PO, IV, IN, smoked)	Euphoria, increased energy, grandiose beliefs, aggression, argumentative, illusions, hallucinations (intact orientation), paranoid ideation, labile mood	↑ HR, ↑ BP, arrhythmias, sweating, N+V, pupillary dilatation, psychomotor agitation, muscular weakness, chest pain, convulsions	Dysphoric mood (must be present), lethargy, psychomotor agitation, craving, increased appetite, insomnia (or hypersomnia), bizarre/unpleasant dreams
Hallucinogens	LSD (lysergic acid diethylamide), magic mushrooms	PO	Anxiety, illusions, hallucinations, depersonalization, derealization, paranoia, ideas of reference, hyperactivity, impulsivity, inattention	↑ HR, palpitations, sweating, tremor, blurred vision, pupillary dilatation, incoordination	n/a
Volatile solvents	Aerosols, paint, glue, petrol	Inhaled	Apathy, lethargy, aggression, impaired attention and judgement, psychomotor retardation	Unsteady gait, diplopia, nystagmus, decreased consciousness, muscle weakness	n/a
Anabolic steroids	Testosterone, androstenedione, danazol	PO, IM	Euphoria, depression, aggression, hyperactivity, mood swings, hallucinations, delusions	Increased muscle mass, reduced fat, acne, male pattern baldness, reduced sperm count/infertility, stunted growth	n/a

Epidemiology and risk factors (Fig. 7.1.1)

- Substance misuse is more common in ♂ at a ratio of **3:1 (♂:♀)**.
- **Cannabis** is the **most consumed** illegal drug, used by **5%** of the population.

Clinical features

- Clinical features vary depending on the drug consumed. Commonly misused substances are **opioids**, **cannabinoids**, **stimulants**, **sedative-hypnotics**, **hallucinogens**, **volatile solvents** and **anabolic steroids**.
- Complications of substance misuse can be divided in physical, psychological and social (*Fig. 7.1.2*).

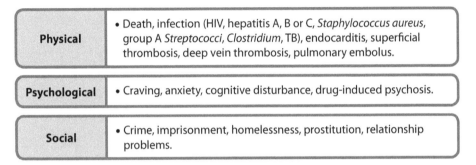

Physical	• Death, infection (HIV, hepatitis A, B or C, *Staphylococcus aureus*, group A *Streptococci*, *Clostridium*, TB), endocarditis, superficial thrombosis, deep vein thrombosis, pulmonary embolus.
Psychological	• Craving, anxiety, cognitive disturbance, drug-induced psychosis.
Social	• Crime, imprisonment, homelessness, prostitution, relationship problems.

Fig. 7.1.2: Physical, psychological and social complications of drug misuse.

Key facts 1: Substance dependence [DRUG PROBLEMS WILL CONTINUE TO HARM]

- Substance dependence describes a syndrome including behavioural, physiological and psychological elements. Patients are physiologically dependent if they show tolerance or withdrawal.
- **≥3** of the following manifestations must have occurred over **1 month**: (1) Strong **Desire (compulsion)** to consume substance; (2) **Preoccupation** with substance use; (3) **Withdrawal state** when substance ingestion is **reduced** or **stopped**; (4) **Impaired ability** to **Control** substance-taking behaviour (e.g. onset, termination or level of use); (5) **Tolerance** to substance, requiring more consumption for desired effect; (6) Persisting with use, despite clear evidence to the **Harmful effects**.

Diagnosis and investigations

Hx The history may be difficult to elicit as people may not be honest about illegal activity (see *Key facts 2*). Obtain a collateral history to help determine the extent of substance misuse.

- 'Have you ever taken any recreational drugs? If so, how often do you take them, and for how long have you done this?', 'How much money do you spend, per week, on drugs?' **(quantity)**
- 'What are the effects when you take the drug?' **(drug effects)**
- 'What impact has the drug had on your life?' **(occupation, relationships, forensic history)**
- 'Do you feel that taking the drug is always at the forefront of your mind?' **(preoccupation)**
- 'Have you ever tried reducing the substance you're taking? Any problems with this?' **(withdrawal)**
- 'Are you able to control your consumption?' **(control)**
- 'Do you recently feel that you have to take more of the drug to get the same effect?' **(tolerance)**
- 'Are you aware of the harmful effects?' **(knowledge of harm)**

Key facts 2: Classes of drugs according to UK law

Class	Examples	Possession	Supply/Production
A	Crack cocaine, cocaine, ecstasy, heroin, LSD, methamphetamine, methadone, magic mushrooms	Up to 7 years in prison and/or unlimited fine	Up to life imprisonment and/or unlimited fine
B	Amphetamines, barbiturates, cannabis, ketamine, methylphenidate	Up to 5 years in prison and/or unlimited fine	Up to 14 years in prison and/or unlimited fine
C	Anabolic steroids, benzodiazepines, khat, gamma-hydroxybutyrate (GHB)	Up to 2 years in prison and/or unlimited fine (excluding anabolic steroids)	Up to 14 years in prison and/or unlimited fine

OSCE tips: History taking in substance misuse

- Substance misuse is often a sensitive issue to ask questions on. As such, in an OSCE you will be awarded marks for **rapport and empathy**, **active listening** and a **non-judgemental attitude**.
- It is useful to divide your history into **current use** (including 'TRAP' [Type, Route, Amount, Pattern] and exploring the signs of dependency, see *Key facts 1*), **risk assessment** (suicide/self-harm as well as IV use/needle sharing), **possible triggers** or stressful life events, **past substance use, physical, psychological** and **social complications** of drugs abuse (e.g. future use), and **coping strategies**.

> **MSE** Dependent upon the drug consumed and whether patient is acutely intoxicated or withdrawing.

NOTE: Perform a **full systems examination** including respiratory, cardiovascular, gastrointestinal and neurological, and a full set of **observations** is required including RR, HR, BP and neurological observations (including GCS).

> **Ix**
> - **Bloods** including: (1) **HIV** screen, **Hep B**, **Hep C** and tuberculosis testing → risk of blood-borne infections is thought to be greater through needle sharing; (2) **U&Es** to check renal function; (3) **LFTs and clotting** to check hepatic function; (4) **Drug levels**.
> - **Urinalysis:** drug metabolites (e.g. cannabis, opioids) can be detected in urine.
> - **ECG** for arrhythmias, **ECHO** if endocarditis suspected (secondary to needle sharing).

> **DDx**
> - **Psychiatric disorders:** Psychosis, mood disorders, anxiety disorders, delirium.
> - **Organic disorders:** Hyperthyroidism, CVA, intracranial haemorrhage, neurological disorders (e.g. cerebellar pathology).

Management (includes NICE guidance)

- A **keyworker** with a **therapeutic alliance** is best placed to offer psychosocial support.
- **Hep B immunization** must be considered for those at risk.
- **Motivational interviewing** to help with controlling the substance misuse and **CBT** (for co-morbid depression or anxiety) may be offered.
- **Contingency management** is a technique that focuses on changing specified behaviours by offering incentives (e.g. financial) for positive behaviours such as abstinence.
- **Supportive help** can be in **housing**, **finance** and **employment**. Help with co-existing **alcohol misuse** and **smoking cessation** should be offered.
- **Self-help groups**, e.g. **Narcotics Anonymous** and **Cocaine Anonymous**.
- Consider the **issue of driving** and review the DVLA guidelines.

Key facts 3: Detoxification vs. maintenance

Detoxification refers to a process in which the effects of the drug are eliminated in a safe manner (a replacement drug is weaned) such that withdrawal symptoms are avoided, in an attempt to attain abstinence. In **maintenance** therapy abstinence is not the priority, rather the aim is to minimize harm (e.g. from IV drug use).

Opioid dependence

- **Biological therapies** include **methadone** (first-line) or **buprenorphine** for **detoxification** AND **maintenance** (see *Key facts 3*).
- **Naltrexone** is recommended for those who were formerly opioid-dependent but have now stopped and are motivated to continue abstinence.
- **Intravenous naloxone** (opioid antagonist) can be used as an **antidote** to opioid overdose.

Self-assessment

A 20-year-old man presents to A&E with a GCS of 10, respiratory depression, and miosis (1 mm pupils). His friends state that the man was seen injecting something intravenously at a party, shortly after which he became unresponsive. He is deeply unresponsive to pain and is unable to give a history. The patient is a known drug user and has track marks on both upper extremities and syringes are found among his belongings.

1. What type of drug is the man most likely to have taken? *(1 mark)*
2. Under what class of drugs would this drug be categorized? *(1 mark)*
3. What antidote should be given to this patient and how is this administered? *(2 marks)*
4. Name four features of drug dependence. *(4 marks)*
5. Name three psychosocial interventions for his long-term management. *(3 marks)*

Answers to self-assessment questions are to be found in *Appendix B*.

Alcohol abuse is the consumption of alcohol at a level sufficient to cause **physical**, **psychiatric** and/or **social harm**. **Binge drinking** is drinking **over twice the recommended level** of alcohol per day, in **one session** (>**8 units** for ♂ and >**6 units** for ♀). **Harmful alcohol use** is defined as **drinking above safe levels** with evidence of **alcohol-related problems** (>**50 units/week** for ♂ and >**35 units/week** for ♀).

Pathophysiology/Aetiology

- Alcohol affects several **neurotransmitter systems** in the brain (e.g. its effect on **GABA** causes **anxiolytic** and **sedative** effects).

- The pleasurable and stimulant effects of alcohol are mediated by a **dopaminergic pathway** in the brain. Repeated, excessive alcohol ingestion sensitizes this pathway and leads to the development of dependence.

- Long-term exposure to alcohol causes adaptive changes in several neurotransmitter systems, including **down-regulation** of **inhibitory neuronal GABA** receptors and **up-regulation** of **excitatory glutamate** receptors, so when alcohol is withdrawn, it results in central nervous system **hyper-excitability**.

- Patients with alcohol-use disorders often experience **craving** (a conscious desire or urge to drink alcohol). This has been linked to **dopaminergic**, **serotonergic**, and **opioid systems** that mediate **positive reinforcement**, and to the **GABA**, **glutamatergic**, and **noradrenergic systems** that mediate **withdrawal**.

- The **social learning theory** suggests that drinking behaviour is modelled on **imitation** of relatives or friends. **Operant conditioning** states that **positive** or **negative reinforcement** from the effects of drinking will either perpetuate or deter drinking habits, respectively.

Key facts 1: Recommended maximum intake of alcohol

MALE ♂	FEMALE ♀
14 units per week	14 units per week

The recommended limits used to be 3–4 units *per day* (males) and 2–3 units *per day* (females). However, guidance changed in January 2016 to 14 units *per week*, with no differentiation between men and women.

Epidemiology and risk factors (*Table 7.2.1*)

- Roughly **25%** of ♂ and **15%** of ♀ drink over the recommended level in the UK.
- Alcohol dependence affects **4%** of people between the ages of **16 and 65** in England.

Table 7.2.1: Risk factors for alcohol abuse

Male	• Males are at **increased risk** of alcohol abuse and have **increased metabolism** of alcohol, thus allowing them to have higher quantities.
Younger adults	• 16.2% among 18–29 year olds; 9.7% among 30–44 year olds have alcohol-related disorders.
Genetics	• **Monozygotic twins** have **higher concordance** rates than dizygotic. Studies show increased risk of dependence in relatives of those affected.
Antisocial behaviour	• Pre-morbid antisocial behaviour has been found to predict alcoholism.

Table 7.2.1: Risk factors for alcohol abuse *(continued)*	
Lack of facial flushing	• The risk of alcoholism is ↓ in individuals who show alcohol-induced facial flushing due to a mutation of gene coding for aldehyde dehydrogenase so that it metabolizes acetaldehyde more slowly. Commoner in some East Asian populations.
Life stressors	• E.g. **Financial problems, marital issues** and **certain occupations** can increase the risk.

Clinical features

• Clinical features vary depending on the alcohol-related disorder.

Alcohol intoxication

• Characterized by **slurred speech, labile affect, impaired judgement** and **poor co-ordination**.
• In severe cases, there may be **hypoglycaemia, stupor** and **coma**.

Alcohol dependence
(Edward and Gross Criteria – 'SAW DRINk')

• **S**ubjective awareness of compulsion to drink.
• **A**voidance or relief of withdrawal symptoms by further drinking (also known as relief drinking).
• **W**ithdrawal symptoms.
• **D**rink-seeking behaviour predominates.
• **R**einstatement of drinking after attempted abstinence.
• **I**ncreased tolerance to alcohol.
• **N**arrowing of drinking repertoire (i.e. a stereotyped pattern of drinking – individuals have fixed as opposed to variable times for drinking, with reduced influence from environmental cues).

Alcohol withdrawal

• Symptoms such as malaise, tremor, nausea, insomnia, transient hallucinations and autonomic hyperactivity occur at 6–12 hours after abstinence. Peak incidence of seizures at 36 hours.

Medical
• **Hepatic:** fatty liver, hepatitis, cirrhosis, hepatocellular carcinoma (*Fig. 7.2.2*). • **Gastrointestinal:** peptic ulcer disease, oesophageal varices, pancreatitis, oesophageal carcinoma. • **Cardiovascular:** hypertension, cardiomyopathy, arrhythmias. • **Haematological:** anaemia, thrombocytopenia. • **Neurological:** seizures, peripheral neuropathy, cerebellar degeneration, Wernicke's encephalopathy, Korsakoff's psychosis, head injury (secondary to falls). • **Obstetrics:** fetal alcohol syndrome.

Psychiatric
• Morbid jealousy. • Self-harm and suicide. • Mood disorders. • Anxiety disorders. • Alcohol-related dementia. • Alcoholic hallucinosis. • Delirium tremens.

Social
• Domestic violence. • Drink driving (See *Key facts 4*). • Employment difficulties. • Financial problems. • Homelessness. • Accidents. • Relationship problems.

Fig. 7.2.1: Negative effects of alcohol consumption.

- The severe end of the spectrum of withdrawal is also termed **delirium tremens** and the peak incidence is at **72 hours** (see *Key facts 2*).
- Alcohol abuse has many **long-term effects** (*Fig. 7.2.1*).

ICD-10 Criteria for alcohol intoxication	ICD-10 Criteria for alcohol withdrawal
A. **General criteria for acute intoxication met:** (1) clear evidence of psychoactive substance use at high dose levels; (2) disturbance in consciousness, cognition, perception or behaviour; (3) not accounted for by medical or mental disorder. B. **Evidence of dysfunctional behaviour:** disinhibition, argumentativeness, aggression, labile mood, impaired attention/concentration, interference with personal functioning. **One** of following signs: unsteady gait, difficulty standing, slurred speech, nystagmus, flushing, ↓ consciousness, conjunctival injection.	A. **General criteria for a withdrawal state met:** (1) clear evidence of recent cessation or reduction of substance after prolonged or high level usage; (2) not accounted for by medical or mental disorder. B. Any **three** of the following: tremor, sweating, nausea/vomiting, tachycardia/↑ BP, headache, psychomotor agitation, insomnia, malaise, transient hallucinations, grand mal convulsions.

Key facts 2: Delirium tremens

- This **withdrawal delirium** develops between **24 hours and one week** after alcohol cessation. Peak incidence of delirium tremens is at **72 hours**.
- Physical illness is a predisposing factor.
- **Dehydration** and **electrolytic disturbances** are a feature.
- It is characterized by:
  - **Cognitive impairment**
  - **Vivid perceptual abnormalities** (hallucinations and/or illusions)
  - **Paranoid delusions**
  - **Marked tremor**
  - **Autonomic arousal** (e.g. tachycardia, fever, pupillary dilatation and increased sweating).
- Medical treatment can be with large doses of **benzodiazepines** (e.g. chlordiazepoxide), **haloperidol** for any psychotic features, and **intravenous Pabrinex**.

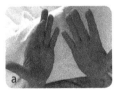 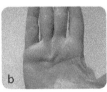

Fig. 7.2.2: Peripheral stigmata of chronic liver disease in alcoholics. (a) palmar erythema; (b) Dupuytren's contracture; (c) spider naevi; (d) gynaecomastia. Other features include clubbing, caput medusa and oesophageal varices.

Diagnosis and investigations

Hx
- See *OSCE tips 2*.
  NOTE: A collateral history is important.

OSCE tips 1: CAGE questionnaire

A useful screening tool for alcohol dependence in an OSCE setting are the **'CAGE' questions**. The patient has a problem if they answer yes to any of the following questions:
- **C** – Have you ever felt you should **Cut** down on your drinking?
- **A** – Have people **Annoyed** you by criticizing your drinking?
- **G** – Have you ever felt **Guilty** about your drinking?
- **E** – Do you ever have a drink early in the morning to steady your nerves or wake you up? (**E**ye opener)

MSE

	Intoxication	Withdrawal
Appearance & Behaviour	Poor co-ordination, secondary injuries (e.g. lacerations), smell of alcohol.	Agitated, sweaty, tremor. May have seizures.
Speech	Slurred.	Confused.
Mood	May be elevated or depressed. Labile affect.	Anxious.
Thought	Variable. Disinhibited.	Paranoid delusions.
Perception	No abnormalities.	Visual hallucinations, illusions.
Cognition	Impaired judgement, reduced concentration.	Delirium, inattention.
Insight	Poor.	Poor.

NOTE: It is important to carry out neurological, cardiovascular and GI examinations (*Fig. 7.2.1*).

OSCE tips 2: Specific alcohol history

1. **Screen for alcohol dependence**
   - See *CAGE questionnaire* above.
2. **Establish drinking pattern and quantity consumed**
   - 'Can you describe what drinks you have in a typical day?'
   - 'How much alcohol do you consume in an average week?' (quantify number of units)
   - 'How much money do you spend on drinking?'
   - 'How often do you consume alcohol?'
   - 'Do you drink steadily or have periods of binge drinking?'
   - 'Is there anything in particular which causes you to drink more?'

OSCE tips 2: Specific alcohol history *(continued)*

3. **Explore features of alcohol dependence**
   - 'When and where do you normally drink?' **(narrowing of drinking repertoire)**
   - 'Do you often feel the urge to drink?' **(compulsive need to drink)**
   - 'Have you noticed that alcohol has less effect on you than it had in the past?' **($\uparrow$ tolerance)**
   - 'Is alcohol the first thing that comes into your mind when planning a social gathering?' **(drink-seeking behaviour predominates)**
   - 'Do you ever feel shaky and anxious when you haven't had a drink?', 'Have you ever tried to give up drinking, if so what happened?' **(withdrawal effects)**
   - 'Do you ever drink to get rid of this feeling?' **(prevention of withdrawal effects)**
4. **Explore possible risk factors**
   - 'Is there any family history of alcohol-related problems?'
   - Explore other risk factors, e.g. financial difficulties, relationship difficulties, etc.
5. **Establish impact**
   - 'Has alcohol affected your mental health?' **(psychiatric impact)**
   - 'Has alcohol affected your medical health?' Ask about alcohol-related disorders, e.g. liver disease, cardiovascular disease, neurological disorders **(physical impact)**
   - 'Has alcohol caused any problems with work, relationships or the law?' **(social impact)**

Ix
- **Bloods** including: blood alcohol level, **FBC** (anaemia), **U&Es** (dehydration, $\downarrow$ urea), **LFTs** including gamma GT (may be $\uparrow$), **blood alcohol concentration**, **MCV** (macrocytosis), **vitamin B$_{12}$/folate/TFTs** (alternative causes of $\uparrow$MCV), **amylase** (pancreatitis), **hepatitis serology**, **glucose** (hypoglycaemia).
- **Alcohol questionnaires:** Alcohol Use Disorders Identification Test (AUDIT), Severity of Alcohol Dependence Questionnaire (SADQ), FAST screening tool (4 items, designed for busy settings).
- **CT head** (if head injury is suspected).
- **ECG** (for arrhythmias).

DDx

Psychiatric disorders:	Medical disorders:
• Psychosis.	• Head injury.
• Mood disorders (including bipolar).	• Cerebral tumour.
• Anxiety disorders.	• Cerebrovascular accident (e.g. stroke).
• Delirium.	

Key facts 3: Neuropsychiatric complications (Wernicke's encephalopathy and Korsakoff's psychosis)

- *Wernicke's encephalopathy:* An **acute encephalopathy** due to **thiamine deficiency**, presenting with **delirium, nystagmus, ophthalmoplegia, hypothermia** and **ataxia**. Requires urgent treatment and may progress to **Korsakoff's psychosis** (AKA amnesic syndrome). Treated with **parenteral thiamine**.
- *Korsakoff's psychosis:* Profound, irreversible **short-term memory loss** with **confabulation** (the unconscious filling of gaps in memory with imaginary events) and **disorientation to time**.

OSCE tips 3: Quantifying the amount of alcohol consumed

- **One unit** of alcohol is defined as a drink containing **10 ml (8g)** of **ethanol.**

  Alcohol units = [strength (alcohol by volume) × volume (ml)] ÷ 1000

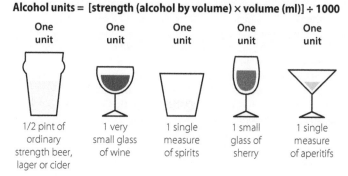

One unit	One unit	One unit	One unit	One unit
1/2 pint of ordinary strength beer, lager or cider	1 very small glass of wine	1 single measure of spirits	1 small glass of sherry	1 single measure of aperitifs

Management (NICE guidance 2011)

See *Fig. 7.2.3* for an overview of the **bio-psychosocial management** of alcohol abuse.

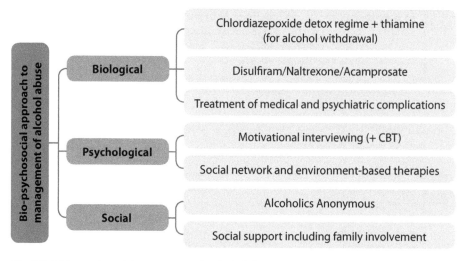

Fig. 7.2.3: Bio-psychosocial management for alcohol abuse.

Key facts 4: Alcohol misuse and driving

- It is the patient's responsibility to contact the **DVLA** if there is alcohol misuse or dependence.
- If at follow-up, you find that the patient has not informed the DVLA, consider first contacting your Medical Defence Union for advice, inform the person in writing of your intended actions so as to give them another opportunity, and if this does not work then contact the DVLA personally.

For alcohol withdrawal

- It is important to recognize signs of alcohol dependence as the withdrawal syndrome is associated with significant morbidity and mortality.

- An alcohol detoxification regime offers controlled withdrawal, and can be carried out in the community or as an inpatient in more severe cases, in order to achieve **abstinence**. **Inpatient** detoxification is recommended in patients at **risk of suicide**, those with **poor social support** or those with a **history of severe withdrawal reactions**.

- **High dose benzodiazepines** (commonly **chlordiazepoxide**) are given initially, and the dose is **tapered down** over 5–9 days (see *Table 7.2.2*).

- Thiamine (Vitamin B$_1$) is also given in order to prevent **Wernicke's encephalopathy**. This can be given **orally** (200–300 mg daily in divided doses) or **intravenously** (in the form of **Pabrinex**).

Table 7.2.2: An example of a chlordiazepoxide regime

DRUG chlordiazepoxide		Time	Day 1 Dose	Day 2 Dose	Day 3 Dose	Day 4 Dose	Day 5 Dose	Day 6 Dose	Day 7 Dose	Day 8 Dose	Day 9 Dose
Dose	**Route**	8	20 mg	20 mg	15 mg	15 mg	10 mg	10 mg	5 mg	5 mg	–
variable	oral	12	20 mg	15 mg	15 mg	10 mg	10 mg	5 mg	5 mg	–	–
Signature		18	20 mg	15 mg	15 mg	10 mg	10 mg	5 mg	5 mg	–	–
		22	20 mg	20 mg	15 mg	15 mg	10 mg	10 mg	5 mg	5 mg	5 mg

For alcohol dependence (long term)

- Pharmacological therapies include:

    1. **Disulfiram:** Works by causing a build-up of acetaldehyde on consumption of alcohol, causing unpleasant symptoms e.g. anxiety, flushing and headache.

    2. **Acamprosate:** Reduces craving by enhancing GABA transmission.

    3. **Naltrexone:** Blocks opioid receptors (antagonist) in the body, thus reducing the pleasurable effects of alcohol.

- Motivational interviewing guides the person into wanting to change (*Fig. 7.2.4*). Motivational interviewing is most effective during the pre-contemplation and contemplation phases.

- CBT can be effective in managing alcohol problems and focuses specifically on alcohol-related beliefs and behaviours.

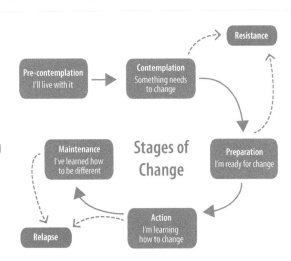

Fig. 7.2.4: 'Stages of change' model.

- Alcoholics Anonymous (AA) is a popular supportive programme for patients who accept that they have a drinking problem. It is a **12-step approach** that utilizes **psychosocial techniques** in order to change behaviour (e.g. social support networks, rewards). Each new member is assigned a 'sponsor' (a supervisor recovering from alcoholism).

General points

- Preventive measures include **raising taxation** on alcohol, **restricted advertising** or **sales**, and more **education** on alcohol issues in schools.
- Prophylactic oral thiamine (50 mg once daily) should be offered to harmful drinkers if they are **malnourished** (or at risk of malnourishment) or have **decompensated liver disease**.

Self-assessment

A 32-year-old man presents for a routine check-up for his blood pressure. He is found to have a BP of 172/88. You notice that he appears unkempt with an obvious odour of alcohol and that his speech is slurred. His concerned partner states she is worried about his drinking which is out of control and that he has been requiring more and more alcohol recently.

1. Aside from ↑ tolerance to alcohol, name four other features of alcohol dependence. *(4 marks)*
2. Name two medical, two psychiatric and two social complications of excess alcohol intake. *(3 marks)*
3. Define delirium tremens and state its five features. *(6 marks)*
4. What is the pharmacological management for alcohol withdrawal? *(2 marks)*

Answers to self-assessment questions are to be found in *Appendix B*.

Chapter 8

Personality disorders

Definition

A **deeply ingrained** and **enduring pattern of inner experience and behaviour** that deviates markedly from expectations in the individual's culture, is **pervasive** and **inflexible**, has an **onset** in **adolescence** or **early adulthood**, is **stable** over time and leads to **distress** or **impairment**.[1]

Pathophysiology/Aetiology

- The cause of personality disorders (PD) involves both **biological** and **environmental** factors (*Table 8.1*).
- **Biological** factors can be **genetic** and **neurodevelopmental** (abnormal cerebral maturation).
- **Environmental** factors encompass both **adverse social circumstances** and **difficult childhood experiences** such as abuse.
- PDs can be classified into **three clusters** assigned **A**, **B** and **C** based on symptoms (*Fig. 8.1*).

Table 8.1: Risk factors for personality disorders	
Society	• Both **low socioeconomic status** and social reinforcement of abnormal behaviour are linked to PDs.
Genetics	• **Monozygotic twin studies** show a **higher concordance rate** for PD than dizygotic studies. Incidence is higher in those with a **positive family history** of PD.
Dysfunctional family	• **Poor parenting** and **parental deprivation** are risks for the development of PD.
Abuse during childhood	• This includes physical, sexual (particularly linked to emotionally unstable PD) and emotional **abuse**, as well as neglect.

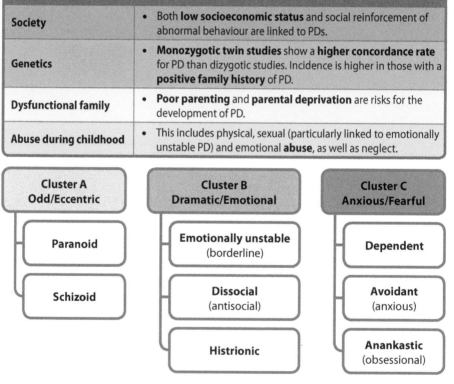

Fig. 8.1: Types of personality disorder based on *ICD-10*.

Epidemiology and risk factors

- **4–13%** of the **adult population** has a PD of at least mild severity.
- **20%** of **GP attendees** who are adults suffer from a PD.
- The most prevalent PD is **dissocial (3%)** followed by **histrionic (2–3%)** and **paranoid (0.5–2.5%)**.

Clinical features

- The clinical features of the **eight specific PDs** classified by *ICD-10* are shown in *Table 8.2*.
- A useful mnemonic for remembering clusters is **WWW**: Cluster A = 'Weird'; Cluster B = 'Wild'; Cluster C = 'Worriers'.

Table 8.2: The features of personality disorders[2]

Cluster A (Weird)

Paranoid 'SUSPECTS'	• Suspicious of others • Unforgiving (bears grudges) • Spouse fidelity questioned • Perceives attack	• Envious (jealous) • Criticism not liked/Cold affect • Trust in others reduced • Self-reference
Schizoid 'DISTANT'	• Detached (flattened) affect • Indifferent to praise or criticism • Sexual drive reduced • Tasks done alone	• Absence of close friends • No emotion (cold) • Takes pleasure in few activities

Cluster B (Wild)

Emotionally unstable (borderline) 'AM SUICIDE'	• Abandonment feared • Mood instability • Suicidal behaviour • Unstable relationships • Intense relationships	• Control of anger poor • Impulsivity • Disturbed sense of self (identity) • Emptiness (chronic)
Dissocial (antisocial) 'CORRUPT'	• Callous • Others blamed • Reckless disregard for safety • Remorseless (lack of guilt)	• Underhanded (deceitful) • Poor planning (impulsive) • Temper/Tendency to violence
Histrionic 'PRAISE'	• Provocative behaviour • Real concern for physical attractiveness • Attention seeking	• Influenced easily • Shallow/Seductive inappropriately • Egocentric (vain)/Exaggerated emotions

Cluster C (Worriers)

Dependent 'RELIANCE'	• Reassurance required • Expressing disagreement is difficult • Lack of self-confidence • Initiating projects is difficult	• Abandonment feared • Needs others to assume responsibility • Companionship sought • Exaggerated fears
Anxious (avoidant) 'CRIES'	• Certainty of being liked needed before becoming involved with people • Restriction to lifestyle in order to maintain security • Inadequacy felt	• Embarrassment potential prevents involvement in new activities • Social inhibition

Table 8.2: The features of personality disorders *(continued)*

Anankastic (obsessional) 'LAW FIRMS'	• Loses point of activity (due to preoccupation with detail) • Ability to complete tasks compromised (due to perfectionism) • Workaholic at the expense of leisure	• Fussy (excessively concerned with minor details) • Inflexible • Rigidity • Meticulous attention to detail • Stubborn

OSCE tips 1: Differentiating between 'Cluster A' PDs and psychotic disorders

'Cluster A' PDs (paranoid and schizoid) may present with similar features to psychotic disorders, e.g. schizophrenia, for instance with suspiciousness, odd beliefs and social withdrawal. The differentiating factor is that hallucinations and true delusions are ABSENT in 'Cluster A' PDs.

Diagnosis and investigations

Hx

- 'How do you think your friends and family would describe your personality?' **(open question)**
- 'Are you ever concerned about other people in your life?', 'Can you rely on friends and family?', 'How do you view your relationship with family?' **(paranoid)**
- 'Do you work well with others?', 'What activities do you enjoy?', 'Would you say you have many close friends?' **(schizoid)**
- 'How would you describe your relationships with the people in your life?', 'Do other people ever say you have a temper?', 'Do you ever feel life is not worth living?', 'Do you have any worries about being alone?' **(emotionally unstable)**
- 'Have you ever got into serious trouble, for instance with the police? If so, was it your fault?', 'Do people ever tell you that you have a temper?', 'Do you like to think things through properly before carrying out an act?' **(dissocial)**
- 'Do you feel that you are easily influenced by your friends?', 'Do you like to be the life and soul of a party?' **(histrionic)**
- 'Is there anything you worry about or fear?', 'Do you struggle to make an important decision?', 'Place yourself on a scale ranging from very shy to confident.' **(dependent)**
- 'Tell me about your social circle', 'Do you ever take risks or partake in brand new activities?', 'Do you feel contented with yourself?' **(anxious)**
- 'Do you feel that you are a perfectionist?', 'Do you spend more time working or relaxing?', 'Do you find you are struggling to meet deadlines at work?' **(anankastic)**
- **A reliable collateral history is imperative:** to determine the course of the symptoms, as well as identifying characteristic features which the patient may not have disclosed.

MSE MSE findings will vary depending on the type of PD and the features associated.

OSCE tips 2: Insight

Patients with PDs often have **no insight** into their psychiatric disorder. It is almost impossible to make a diagnosis of personality disorder without taking a **reliable collateral history** to elicit the pervasiveness and stability of the presentation. You need to complete a detailed personal and social history to understand the impact of the disorder on relationships, friendships and occupation.

Ix
- **Questionnaires:** e.g. Personality Diagnostic Questionnaire, Eysenck Personality Questionnaire.
- **Psychological testing:** Minnesota Multiphasic Personality Inventory (MMPI).
- **CT head/MRI:** to rule out organic causes of personality change such as frontal lobe tumours and intracranial bleeds.

DDx
- **Mood disorders:** Mania, depression.
- **Psychotic disorders:** Schizophrenia, schizoaffective disorder.
- **Substance misuse.**

Management (includes NICE guidance 2009)

- See *Fig. 8.2* for the principles of managing PD.
- Co-morbid **psychiatric illness** and **substance misuse** are common in patients with PD. Their recognition and treatment are essential.
- **Risk assessment** is crucial, particularly in cases of **emotionally unstable PD**, where patients may be suicidal. Potential **stressors** that induce crises should be identified and reduced.
- Several **psychosocial interventions** exist in the treatment of PD.
- **Pharmacological management** will not resolve the PD, but may be used to **control symptoms. Low-dose antipsychotics** for ideas of reference, impulsivity and intense anger. **Antidepressants** may be useful in emotionally unstable personality disorder. **Mood stabilizers** can also be given. All of these are off-licence indications for prescribing.
- Give the patient a **written crisis plan**. At times of crisis, if dangerous and violent or if there is a suicide risk consider the **Crisis Resolution Team** and detention under the **Mental Health Act**.
- The management of people with PDs **can be outlined using** the **bio-psychosocial approach** (*Table 8.3*).

Identify and treat co-morbid **mental health disorders**

Treat any co-existing **substance misuse**

Help patient to deal with situations that **provoke problem behaviours or traits**

Provide **general support** to **reduce tension** and **anxieties**

Give **support and reassurance** to **family** and friends

Fig. 8.2: Main principles in managing PD.

Table 8.3: Bio-psychosocial management of personality disorders		
Biological	**Psychological**	**Social**
1. **Atypical antipsychotics** may be used in the short term for transient psychotic periods in certain PDs (e.g. paranoid PD). 2. **Mood stabilizers** can be used in emotionally unstable PD for symptoms such as mood instability and aggression. 3. Small role for **antidepressants**.	1. **Cognitive behavioural therapy.** 2. **Psychodynamic psychotherapy –** which may be individual or group. 3. **Dialectical behavioural therapy** – emphasis placed on developing coping strategies to improve impulse control and reduce self-harm in emotionally unstable PD.	1. **Support groups.** 2. **Substance misuse services.** 3. Assistance with social problems (e.g. housing, finance and employment). 4. Help to access education, voluntary work, meaningful occupation and work.

Self-assessment

A 34-year-old man presents feeling suicidal with a background of numerous acts of deliberate self-harm. He has a turbulent relationship with his girlfriend but tells you he plans to propose to her later that same day. He has been arrested on several occasions for attacking rival supporters at football matches. He reports a difficult childhood, having been sexually abused by his step-father.

1. What is the most likely personality disorder? *(1 mark)*
2. Name six other personality disorders based on the ICD-10 criteria. *(3 marks)*
3. What are the features of antisocial personality disorder? *(3 marks)*
4. Highlight three psychological interventions for personality disorders. *(3 marks)*

Answers to self-assessment questions are to be found in *Appendix B*.

[1] *Diagnostic and Statistical Manual of the American Psychiatric Association*, 4th Ed. American Psychiatric Association. Washington, DC, USA.
[2] Adapted from 'Mnemonics for DSM-IV Personality Disorders', Pinkofsky, H.B., *Psychiatric Services* (1997), **48:** 9.

Chapter 9

Suicide and self-harm

Deliberate self-harm

Definition

Deliberate self-harm (DSH) refers to an **intentional act** of **self-poisoning** or **self-injury** (*Fig. 9.1.1*), **irrespective of the motivation** or apparent purpose of the act. It is usually an expression of **emotional distress**.

> • Cutting, burning, hanging, stabbing, swallowing objects, shooting, jumping from heights or in front of vehicles
>
> **Methods of self-injury**

> • Medication (prescribed or OTC), illicit drugs, household substances (e.g. washing liquid), plant material
>
> **Methods of self-poisoning**

Fig. 9.1.1: Methods of self-harm.

Pathophysiology/Aetiology

- The aetiology of DSH is largely **environmental** (see *Table 9.1.1* and *OSCE tips*).

Epidemiology and risk factors (*Table 9.1.1*)

- DSH affects **2 in 1000** people in the UK.
- It is more common in ♀ at a ratio of 1.5:1, but this varies greatly with age.
- DSH is more common in **adolescents and young adults**. Incidence peaks in ♀ aged **15–19 years**, and in ♂ aged **20–24 years**.
- It is **20–30 times** more common than **suicide**.
- The **rate of suicide** in people who have self-harmed **increases** to between **50–100** times greater than that of the suicide rate in the general population.

Table 9.1.1: Risk factors for deliberate self-harm (DSH largely comes via self-poisoning)

Divorced/single/living alone
Severe life stressors
Harmful drug/alcohol use
Less than 35 (age)
Chronic physical health problems
Violence (domestic) or childhood maltreatment
Socioeconomic disadvantage
Psychiatric illness, e.g. depression, psychosis

Clinical features

- DSH can take the form of:
  - Self-poisoning in the form of overdose.
  - Self-injury in the form of cutting, burning, slashing.
- In the UK, **90%** of DSH cases are a result of **drug overdose**. Commonly ingested medications are **non-opioid analgesics** including paracetamol and salicylates (aspirin), **anxiolytics** (including benzodiazepines), and **antidepressants** (self-harmers are commonly depressed).
- **10%** of DSH cases are due to **self-injury**. Common locations for cuts with razors or glass are the forearms and wrists (*Fig. 9.1.2*).

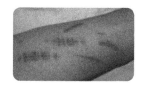

Fig. 9.1.2: Self-injury in the form of cutting.

- Other less common methods of self-injury include jumping in front of moving vehicles or from great heights and attempting to drown oneself (*Fig. 9.1.1*).
- About half the men and a quarter of women who self-harm have taken alcohol in the 6 hours prior to the act, indicating that alcohol is a key risk factor.
- The two commonest complications of DSH: (1) **Permanent scarring of skin** and **damage to tendons** and **nerves** as a result of self-cutting. (2) **Acute liver failure** due to paracetamol overdose.

Diagnosis and investigations

Hx
- What were their **intentions** before and during the act? **(intention)**
- Does the patient now wish to die? **(suicidal ideation)**
- What are the **current problems** in their life? **(severe life stressors)**
- Is there a **psychiatric disorder**? **(psychiatric illness)**
- **Collateral history** from relatives, friends or the GP is important.
- For further details see *Section 9.2*, Risk assessment, *OSCE tips 1–3*.

OSCE tips: Motives behind deliberate self-harm (ask about these) – '**DRIPS**'

- **Death wish:** genuine **wish to die**.
- **Relief:** seeking unconsciousness or pain as a means of **temporary relief** and escape from problems.
- **Influencing others:** trying to **influence another person** to change their views or behaviour (e.g. making a spouse feel guilty for not caring enough).
- **Punishment:** to **punish oneself**.
- **Seeking attention:** trying to get **help** or **seek attention** (expression of emotional distress).

MSE General points on assessment of the patient who has self-harmed:
- Obvious **self-inflicted injuries** may be seen. The patient may be **tearful** or exhibit **signs of neglect**. **Behaviour** may reflect an underlying mental disorder (depression, schizophrenia).
- Thoughts may include feelings of **guilt**, **worthlessness** or **helplessness**.
- **Hallucinations** may be present in cases of **schizophrenia** and **depression with psychosis** where DSH is triggered by **command hallucinations**.
- **Concentration** is often **impaired** and **insight can vary**.

Ix
- **Bloods** including: **Paracetamol levels** (accurate between 4 and 15 hours after ingestion), **salicylate levels** if suspected overdose, **U&Es** (renal function), **LFTs and clotting** (synthetic hepatic function).
- **Urinalysis** for possible toxicological analysis.
- **CT head** if an intracranial cause for altered consciousness is suspected (in self-poisoning).
- **Lumbar puncture** if intracranial infection (e.g. meningitis) suspected (in self-poisoning).

> **DDx** **For self-poisoning:** Head trauma, intracranial haemorrhage, intracranial infection (e.g. meningitis, encephalitis), metabolic abnormalities (e.g. hypoglycaemia), liver disease.
> **For self-injury:** Clotting disorders (causing significant bruising or bleeding).
> **NOTE:** Investigations and differential diagnoses are dependent upon the method of self-harm.

Management (includes NICE guidance)

The **bio-psychosocial management** of self-harm is outlined below:

- Biological: Includes treating any overdose with the appropriate **antidote** (see *Key facts*) and **suturing** (and anti-tetanus treatment if appropriate) for deep lacerations.
- Psychological: Includes **counselling** and **CBT** for underlying **depressive illness**. **Psychodynamic psychotherapy** may be appropriate if the individual has a **personality disorder**. However, this is a long term treatment and needs appropriate assessment.
- Social: **Social services input** and **voluntary organizations** (e.g. the Samaritans, Mind).

General points (Fig. 9.1.3)

- **Risk assessment is mandatory** as there is an immediate risk of suicide and risk of repeat acts of self-harm. Need for hospitalization should be assessed ± use of the **MHA** Section 2.
- There is often involvement of the Crisis team in the community as an alternative to hospital admission (see *Chapter 1*, Introduction to psychiatry).
- If the patient refuses medical treatment for the consequences of self-harm (e.g. acute liver failure, deep lacerations) a **mental capacity assessment** will be required.
- Treat any **underlying psychiatric illness** with medication and/or psychological therapies.
- **Consider safety in overdose of antidepressants** for co-morbid depression. TCAs are most dangerous as they can cause arrhythmias and convulsions in overdose.
- **Psychosocial assessment** is required. Many patients have personal, relationship or social problems for which they can be offered help (e.g. counselling and social service input).
- Ensure that the patient is **followed up** within 48 hours of discharge.
- **NOTE:** that approximately **1 in 6 people** who attend A&E following an act of self-harm will self-harm again **within a year**.

Acute management	Manage high suicide risk	Treat any psychiatric disorder	Enable patient to resolve any difficulties that led to the DSH	Enable patient to manage future crises
Specific antidotes. Suturing. Surgical input for complex wounds.	Full risk assessment. Consider inpatient psychiatric assessment (±MHA).	For instance antidepressants or CBT for depression.	Manage psychosocial needs. Refer to drug/alcohol services if appropriate. Offer financial and occupational rehabillitation advice.	Arrange for follow-up. Offer written and verbal information. Remove access to means of DSH (e.g. prescribe limited supply of meds at any one time).

Fig. 9.1.3: Principles behind managing deliberate self-harm.

Key facts: Antidotes to overdose

Drug	Antidote
Paracetamol	**N-Acetylcysteine**
Opiates	**Naloxone**
Benzodiazepines	**Flumazenil**
Warfarin	**Vitamin K**
Beta-blockers	**Glucagon**
TCAs (e.g. amitriptyline)	**Sodium bicarbonate**
Organophosphates	**Atropine**

- **Activated charcoal:** for the majority of drugs taken in overdose, early use of activated charcoal (within one hour of ingestion) can prevent or reduce absorption of the drug.
- **TOXBASE** can be viewed for information on rarer poisons. The UK **National Poisons Information Service** (NPIS) can also be contacted for further information.

Self-assessment

A 19-year-old female presents to A&E with her boyfriend who states that she has taken a mixed overdose following a disagreement. The boyfriend had received a distressed phone call from the patient prior to her taking the overdose, stating that she loved him and couldn't stand them constantly arguing. He rushed to her apartment 30 minutes ago, only to find her unconscious with an empty bottle of vodka and empty packets of paracetamol and sertraline next to her.

1. Name three risk factors of deliberate self-harm. *(3 mark)*
2. Give three motives behind why people may self-harm. *(3 marks)*
3. What would be your *immediate* management of a paracetamol overdose? *(2 marks)*
4. What is the major complication of paracetamol overdose? *(1 mark)*
5. Three further questions to assess whether the act was a serious attempt at suicide? *(3 marks)*

Answers to self-assessment questions are to be found in *Appendix B*.

- **Suicide:** A fatal act of self-harm initiated with the intention of ending one's own life.
- **Attempted suicide:** The act of intentionally trying to take one's own life with the primary aim of dying, but failing to succeed in this endeavour.
- **Risk assessment:** In a psychiatric context, it is assessing the risk of self-harm, suicide and/or risk to others.

Pathophysiology/Aetiology

- The risk of someone committing suicide is increased by certain risk factors and reduced by certain protective factors (*Fig. 9.2.1*).

Protective factors		Risk factors
Children at home, pregnancy, strong religious beliefs or spiritual belief that suicide is immoral, strong social support, positive coping skills, positive therapeutic relationship, supportive living arrangements, life satisfaction, fear of the physical act of suicide, fear of disapproval by society, responsibility for others, hope for the future.	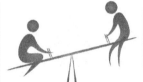	• See *Tables 9.2.1* and *9.2.2*, and *OSCE tips 1*.

OSCE tips 1: Mnemonic for suicide risk factors (**'I'M A SAD PERSON'**)

Institutionalized, Mental health disorders, Alone (lack of social support), Sex (male), Age (middle aged), Depression, Previous attempts, Ethanol use, Rational thinking lost, Sickness, Occupation (see *Table 9.2.2*), No job (unemployed)

Fig. 9.2.1: An imbalance between risk factors and protective factors predisposes to suicide.

Epidemiology and risk factors (*Tables 9.2.1* and *9.2.2*)

- Suicide is the **13th** leading cause of death worldwide, with about **1 million deaths every year** due to self-inflicted violence.
- In 2012, in the **UK** there were **18.2** ♂ suicides **per 100 000 population**, and **5.2** ♀ suicides **per 100 000 population**.
- The most common methods of suicide are **hanging**, **strangulation** and **suffocation** (**58%** of ♂ suicides and **36%** of ♀ suicides), followed by **poisoning** (**43%** of ♀ suicides and **20%** of ♂ suicides).

Table 9.2.1: Clinical risk factors of suicide

History of DSH or attempted suicide	• The rate of suicide in people who have self-harmed increases and is **50–100** times greater than in the general population.
Psychiatric illness	• Including **depression, schizophrenia, substance misuse, alcohol abuse** and **personality disorder**.
Childhood abuse	• History of childhood **sexual** or **physical** abuse.
Family history	• **Family history of suicide or suicide attempt** in first-degree relatives increases the risk.
Medical illness	• Physically **disabling, painful** or **terminal** illness.

Table 9.2.2: Socio-demographic risk factors of suicide

Male gender	• Males are **3x** more likely than females. Male suicide attempts are more likely to be **violent** and therefore successful.
Age	• Highest in the age group **40** to **44** in **men**.
Employment and financial status	• Those **unemployed** and who have **low socioeconomic** status are at higher risk.
Occupation	• **Vets, doctors, nurses** and **farmers** are at higher risk of suicide.
Access to lethal means	• The most lethal means of suicide are **firearms**, followed by **hanging, strangling**, and **suffocation**.
Social support	• **Low social support, living alone, institutionalized**, e.g. prisons, soldiers.
Marital status	• Those that are **single, widowed, seperated** or **divorced**.
Recent life crisis	• e.g. Bereavement, family breakdown.

Clinical features

Individuals who are suicidal usually have a number of characteristics, including the following:

- **Preoccupation with death:** Thoughts, fantasies, ruminations and preoccupations with death, particularly self-inflicted death.
- **Sense of isolation and withdrawal from society.**
- **Emotional distance** from others.
- **Distraction and lack of pleasure:** Often are 'in their own world' and suffer from anhedonia.
- **Focus on the past:** They dwell on past losses and defeats and anticipate no future; they voice the notion of Beck's cognitive triad (see *Section 3.2*, Depressive disorder) that the world would be better off without them.
- **Feelings of hopelessness and helplessness.**

Diagnosis and investigations

Hx
- See *OSCE tips 2 and 3*.
- A **collateral history** may provide valuable information.

MSE See *OSCE tips 3*.

Ix
- Medical investigations according to the method, e.g. drug levels (see *Section 9.1, Deliberate self-harm*).
- Questionnaires - **Tool for Assessment of Suicide Risk (TASR),** Beck Suicide Intent Scale.
- Suicide can be confirmed by **post-mortem**.

OSCE tips 2: Determining the risk of suicide following DSH '**Note: Planned Attempts Are Very Frightening!**' (The following ↑ risk).

1. **N**ote left behind: usually written.
2. **P**lanned attempt of suicide.
3. **A**ttempts to avoid discovery.
4. **A**fterwards help was not sought.
5. **V**iolent method.
6. **F**inal acts: sorting out finances, writing a will.

DDx
- Self-harm (for attempted suicide).

Key facts: Self-harm vs. suicide

Suicide	Self-harm
More common in **males**	More common in **females**
Risk **increases with age**	More common in **young people**
Act may be **planned meticulously**	Act is **impulsive**
Act is more often **violent**	Usually in form of **overdose or cutting**
Physical and **psychiatric illness** is common	**Physical** and **psychiatric illness** is less common

OSCE tips 3: Risk assessment

1. **Exploring suicidal ideation:**
   - 'How do you feel about your future?'
   - 'Do you feel that life is worth living?'
   - 'Have you ever thought about taking your own life?'
2. **Exploring suicide intent:** (see *OSCE tips 2*)
   - What precipitated the attempt? Was it planned?
   - What method did they use?
   - Was a suicide note left? Did they make any other preparations before acting? e.g. writing a will.
   - Was the patient intoxicated with drugs or alcohol?

- Was the patient alone?
- Were there precautions taken to avoid discovery (e.g. they waited until the house was empty, locked doors, timed so that intervention would be highly unlikely)?
- Did the patient think that they were certain to die even if they received medical attention?
- What was the degree of premeditation? How long had they been contemplating suicide for? What plans had they made before acting?
- Did the patient seek help after the attempt or were they found and brought in by someone else?
- How does the patient feel about it now? Do they regret it or do they wish that they had succeeded?
- How do they feel about being found? Are they relieved or are they angry?

3. **Exploring risk factors:**
   - 'Is there anything in particular that is making you feel this way?', 'Can you tell me about it?' (stress)
   - 'Have you ever tried anything like this before?', 'Can you tell me about it?' (previous suicide attempts)
   - 'Are you aware if you are suffering from any mental health illness?' (psychiatric illness)
   - 'Do you have any health problems that are bothering you at the moment?' (medical illness)
   - 'Is there any family history of suicide, attempted suicide or self-harm?' (family history)

4. **Perform mental state examination:**
   May indicate signs of underlying psychiatric disorder (usually depression):
   - **Appearance & behaviour:** e.g. dishevelled, unkempt and unclean clothing, evidence of suicidal behaviour, such as wrist lacerations and neck rope burns.
   - **Mood:** Usually low mood and a flat affect.
   - **Thoughts:** May have delusions about the benefits of suicide (e.g. family will be better off), obsession with taking his or her own life.
   - **Perception** - Possibly second person auditory command hallucinations telling the patient to kill oneself in psychotic depression or schizophrenia.

5. **Explore protective factors:** (see *Fig. 9.2.1*)
   - 'Is there anything that would stop you from carrying out this act?' What are the positive things in their life? (general protective factors)
   - 'Do you have someone to confide in, close family or friends?', 'Who do you live with?', 'Do you have company at home?' (establishing social support or lack of)

6. **Explore risk *to* others (including children) and risk *from* others:**
   - 'Do you ever have thoughts of harming others?'
   - Patients may have children/relatives that are in danger: 'Do you have close contact with any children?' Document the child's name, DOB, place of residence and enquire as to the nature of the relationship.
   - 'Do you ever feel threatened or at risk from others?'

7. **Formulate management plan:**
   - Determine whether the patient is low, medium or high risk and formulate a management plan accordingly, depending on the degree of planning, severity of the attempt and ongoing concerns about risk (see *Management section*).

Management

- **Ensure safety:** Immediate action should include removing means for suicide and ensuring the safety of the patient and others.

- Patients who have attempted suicide and failed, should be **medically stabilized,** e.g. management of drug overdose or treatment of physical injury.

- **Risk assessment:** The risk of further suicide should then be assessed. People with a high degree of suicidal intent, specific plans, or chosen methods (particularly if lethal) should be assigned a higher level of risk (see *OSCE tips 3*).

- **Admission to hospital** (or observation in a safe place) is generally indicated if individuals pose a high and immediate risk of suicide. The **Mental Health Act** might be required if the patient refuses help and there is evidence of a mental illness.

- **Referral to secondary care** (see *OSCE tips 4*).

- **Psychiatric treatment:** Depression or psychosis should be detected and treated accordingly.

- Involvement of the **Crisis Resolution and Home Treatment team** to provide support immediately following discharge can be instrumental.

- **Outpatient and community treatment** may be more suitable for patients with chronic suicidal ideation but no history of previous significant suicide attempts. For this to succeed, a strong support network and easy access to outpatient and community facilities are required.

- **Prevention strategies** (*Fig. 9.2.2*).

> **OSCE tips 4:** When to refer to secondary care for patient at risk of suicide 'SUSPicious'
>
> Is usually considered if: (1) **S**uicidal ideation clearly stated; (2) **U**nderlying psychiatric illness is severe; (3) **S**ocial support (lack of); (4) **P**resentation change for an individual who has repeatedly self-harmed.

Individual suicide prevention strategies	• **Detect and treat psychiatric disorders.** • **Urgent hospitilization** under the **Mental Health Act**. • Involvement of the **Crisis Resolution and home treatment team**.

Population level suicide prevention strategies	• **Public education** and discussion. • **Reducing access to means of suicide**, e.g. encouraging patients to dispose of unwanted tablets, safer prescribing, safety rails at high places. • **Easy, rapid access to psychiatric care** or support groups, e.g. Samaritans (who provide emergency 24 hour support). • **Decreasing societal stressors**, e.g. unemployment and domestic violence. • **Reducing substance misuse.**

Fig. 9.2.2: Individual vs. population suicide prevention strategies.

Self-assessment

A 75-year-old man in a rural village presents to his GP with a 2-week history of constipation, headache, and fatigue. He has a past medical history of ischaemic heart disease and insulin dependent diabetes. He is the primary carer for his wife, who has recently been diagnosed with Alzheimer's disease. Upon further questioning, he admits to feelings of low mood, hopelessness, and persistent suicidal ideation. He feels overwhelmed by the burden of being his wife's carer. He has made vague suicide plans but is worried about how his death would affect his wife's care.

1. What risk factors of suicide does he possess? *(3 marks)*
2. Give four other risk factors of suicide. *(2 marks)*
3. What protective factor of suicide does he possess? *(1 mark)*
4. How should he be managed? *(3 marks)*
5. Give two ways suicide can be prevented on a population level. *(2 marks)*

Answers to self-assessment questions are to be found in *Appendix B*.

Chapter 10

Old age psychiatry

10.1 Delirium

Definition

Delirium is an **acute**, **transient**, **global organic disorder** of CNS functioning resulting in **impaired consciousness** and **attention**. There are different types of delirium: **hypoactive**, **hyperactive** and **mixed** depending on the clinical presentation (*Fig. 10.1.1*).

Hypoactive (40%)
- Lethargy, ↓ motor activity, apathy and sleepiness.
- It is the **most common** type of delirium but often goes unrecognized.
- Can be confused with depression.

Hyperactive (25%)
- Agitation, irritability, restlessness and aggression.
- Hallucinations and delusions prominent.
- May be confused with functional psychoses.

Mixed (35%)
- Both hypo- and hyperactive subtypes co-exist and therefore there are signs of both.

Fig. 10.1.1: Subtypes of delirium.

Pathophysiology/Aetiology

- Delirium has a number of causes (see *Table 10.1.1*); however, most causes of delirium are **multifactorial**, each of which may be important at different time points of the illness. The causes can be remembered using the mnemonic 'HE IS NOT MAAD'.

Table 10.1.1: Causes of delirium ('HE IS NOT MAAD')	
Hypoxia	Respiratory failure, myocardial infarction, cardiac failure, pulmonary embolism.
Endocrine	Hyperthyroidism, hypothyroidism, hyperglycaemia, hypoglycaemia, Cushing's.
Infection	Pneumonia, UTI, encephalitis, meningitis.
Stroke and other intracranial events	Stroke, raised ICP, intracranial haemorrhage, space-occupying lesions, head trauma, epilepsy (post-ictal), intracranial infection.
Nutritional	↓ Thiamine, ↓ nicotinic acid, ↓ vitamin B_{12}.
Others	Severe pain, sensory deprivation (for example leaving the person without spectacles or hearing aids), relocation (such as moving people with impaired cognition to unfamiliar environments), sleep deprivation.
T**heatre (post-operative period)**	Anaesthetic, opiate analgesics and other post-operative complications.

Table 10.1.1: Causes of delirium (' ') (continued)	
etabolic	Hypoxia, electrolyte disturbance (e.g. hyponatraemia), hypoglycaemia, hepatic impairment, renal impairment.
bdominal	Faecal impaction, malnutrition, urinary retention, bladder catheterization.
lcohol	Intoxication, withdrawal (delirium tremens).
rugs	Benzodiazepines, opioids, anticholinergics, anti-parkinsonian medications, steroids.

OSCE tips 1: Medical sieves!

Since there are numerous causes for delirium work through the list systematically by always thinking of the **most common** causes first, e.g. infection (UTI is very common in the elderly).

Epidemiology and risk factors (Table 10.1.2)

- Delirium occurs in about **15–20%** of all general admissions to hospital.
- Delirium is the **most common** complication of hospitalization in the **elderly population**.
- Up to **two-thirds** of delirium cases occur in inpatients with **pre-existing dementia**.
- **15%** of >65s are delirious **on admission** to hospital.

Table 10.1.2: Risk factors for delirium	
Older age ≥65	Multiple co-morbidities
Dementia	Physical frailty
Renal impairment	Male sex
Sensory impairment	Previous episodes
Recent surgery	Severe illness (e.g. CCF)

Clinical features ('DELIRIUM')

Delirium has an **acute onset** and takes a **fluctuating course** (often worse at night). Other features include:

- **D**isordered thinking: Slowed, irrational, incoherent thoughts.
- **E**uphoric, **fearful**, **depressed** or **angry**.
- **L**anguage impaired: Rambling speech, repetitive and disruptive.

ICD-10 Criteria for the diagnosis of delirium

- **Impairment** of **consciousness** and **attention**
- **Global disturbance** in **cognition**
- **Psychomotor disturbance**
- **Disturbance** of **sleep-wake cycle**
- **Emotional disturbances.**

- **I**llusions, **delusions** (transient persecutory or delusions of misidentification) and **hallucinations** (usually tactile or visual).
- **R**eversal of sleep-wake pattern: i.e. may be tired during day and hyper-vigilant at night.
- **I**nattention: Inability to focus, clouding of consciousness.
- **U**naware/disoriented: Disoriented to time, place or person.
- **M**emory deficits.

Key facts: Delirium vs. dementia

	Delirium	Dementia
Sleep-wake cycle	Disrupted	Usually normal
Attention	Markedly reduced	Normal/reduced
Arousal	Increased/decreased	Usually normal
Autonomic features	Abnormal	Normal
Duration	Hours to weeks	Months to years
Delusions	Fleeting	Complex
Course	Fluctuating	Stable/slowly progressive
Consciousness level	Impaired	No impairment
Hallucinations	Common (especially visual)	Less common
Onset	Acute/subacute	Chronic
Psychomotor activity	Usually abnormal	Usually normal

OSCE tips 2: Beware of missing hypoactive delirium!

Delirium may be unrecognized by doctors and nurses in two-thirds of people. Healthcare professionals often do not recognize delirium and may misdiagnose hypoactive delirium as depression. Remember to always consider delirium in a person, particularly an elderly person who is apathetic, quiet or withdrawn.

Diagnosis and investigations

NOTE: Before or during a history, a thorough physical examination should be performed: **ABC** (**A**irway/**B**reathing/**C**irculation), **conscious level** (use AVPU or GCS) and **vital signs**, e.g. oxygen saturations, pulse, blood pressure, temperature, capillary blood glucose. **Nutritional** and **hydration status**, **cardiovascular examination**, **respiratory examination**, **abdominal examination** (check for urinary retention and rectal exam for faecal impaction), **neurological examination** (including speech).

Hx
- **Much of the history may be collateral** as obtaining the history from the patient may prove very difficult.
- Identify rate of onset and course of the confusion.
- Any symptoms of underlying cause, e.g. symptoms of infection or of intracranial pathology?
- Having an understanding of their premorbid mental state is important.
- Are they hypo-alert or hyper-alert?
- Do they have hypersensitivity to sound and light?
- Is there any perceptual disturbance (misidentification, illusions and hallucinations)?
- Take a thorough drug history and a full alcohol history.

MSE	Appearance & Behaviour	Hypo- or hyper-alert. Agitated, aggressive, purposeless behaviour.
	Speech	Incoherent, rambling.
	Mood	Low mood, irritable or anxious. Mood is often labile.
	Thought	Confused, ideas of reference, delusions.
	Perception	Illusions, hallucinations (mainly visual), misinterpretations.
	Cognition	Disoriented, impaired memory, reduced concentration/attention.
	Insight	Poor.

Ix

1. **Routine investigations: Urinalysis** (UTI); **Bloods: FBC** (infection); **U&Es** (electrolyte disturbance); **LFTs** (alcoholism, liver disease); **calcium** (hypercalcaemia); **glucose** (hypo-/hyperglycaemia); **CRP** (infection/inflammation); **TFTs** (hyperthyroidism); **B$_{12}$, folate, ferritin** (nutritional deficiencies); **ECG** (cardiac abnormalities, acute coronary syndrome); **CXR** (chest infection); **Infection screen: blood culture** (sepsis) and **urine culture** (UTI).

2. **Investigations based on history/examination: ABG** (hypoxia), **CT head** (head injury, intracranial bleed, CVA), and you may consider **lumbar puncture** (meningitis), **EEG** (epilepsy).

3. **Diagnostic questionnaire** (helps with diagnosis but also monitoring):
   - **Abbreviated Mental Test (AMT):** A quick easy tool (see *OSCE tips 3*).
   - **Confusion Assessment Method (CAM):** Usually performed after AMT (see *OSCE tips 3*).
   - **Mini-Mental State Examination (MMSE).**

DDx

- **Dementia.**
- **Mood disorders:** depression or mania (bipolar).
- **Late onset schizophrenia.**
- **Dissociative disorders.**
- **Hypothyroidism** and **hyperthyroidism** (may mimic hypo- and hyperactive delirium respectively).

OSCE tips 3: Abbreviated Mental Test (AMT) and Confusion Assessment Method (CAM)

Abbreviated Mental Test	Confusion Assessment Method
1. Age? (1) 2. Time to the nearest hour? (1) 3. Recall address at end: '42 West Street' (1) 4. 'What year is it?' (1) 5. 'Where are you right now?' (1) 6. Identify two people. (1) 7. 'What is your date of birth?' (1) 8. 'Date of First World War?' (1) 9. 'Who is the current monarch?' (1) 10. 'Count backwards from 20 to 1.' (1) **≥8 → cognitive impairment unlikely.**	The Confusion Assessment tool (CAM) involves assessing a patient for four features. The diagnosis involves the presence of **1 and 2 + *either* 3 or 4**: 1. **Acute onset and fluctuating course.** 2. **Inattention** (e.g. using the serial 7s test where 7 is subtracted from 100 and then 7 is taken from each remainder, i.e. 100, 93, 86, 79, 72…). 3. **Disorganized thinking** (e.g. incoherent speech). 4. **Alteration in consciousness.**

Management (*Fig. 10.1.2, includes NICE guidance 2010*)

Treat the underlying cause

- Treat any infections. Correct any electrolyte disturbances.
- Stop any potential offending drugs.
- Laxatives for faecal impaction or temporary catheterization for urinary retention. Give analgesia if required.

Reassurance and re-orientation

- Reassure patients to reduce anxiety and disorientation.
- Patients should be reminded of the time, place, day and date regularly.

Provide appropriate environment

- Quiet, well-lit side room.
- Consistency in care and staff.
- Reassuring nursing staff.
- Encourage presence of friend or family member.
- Optimize sensory acuity, e.g. glasses, well-lit room, orientation aids (clock, calendar).

Managing disturbed, violent or distressed behaviour

- Encourage oral intake and pay attention to continence.
- Verbal and non-verbal de-escalation techniques (e.g. redirection).
- Oral low-dose haloperidol (0.5–4 mg), or olanzapine (2.5–10 mg).
- Avoid benzodiazepines (unless delirium due to alcohol withdrawal).
- Referral to a Care of the Elderly Consultant may be appropriate.

Fig. 10.1.2: Overview of the management of delirium.

OSCE tips 4: Medications are not the answer

Antipsychotics and benzodiazepines are never first-line for managing delirium and unfortunately this is a misconception amongst many clinicians. Treating the underlying cause, providing reassurance and re-orientation and an appropriate environment are the main means for treating delirium as recommended by *NICE guidelines*. Low dose antipsychotics should only be used as a last resort in cases of violent or severely distressed behaviour and when other ways of calming the patient have failed.

Self-assessment

You are bleeped in the middle of the night by a nurse who reports that an 83-year-old man has become disturbed and distressed two days after his abdominal surgery. The patient has been pulling out his cannulas, shouting, repeatedly getting out of bed despite being unsteady, and has been aggressive towards staff. You suspect the patient is suffering from delirium post-operatively.

1. Name four differences between delirium and dementia. *(4 marks)*
2. Name six common causes of delirium. *(3 marks)*
3. What routine investigations would you perform on this patient? *(5 marks)*
4. Name two tools you can use to test his cognition. *(2 marks)*
5. How should this patient be managed? *(5 marks)*

Answers to self-assessment questions are to be found in *Appendix B.*

Dementia

Dementia is a syndrome of generalized decline of **memory**, **intellect** and **personality**, without impairment of **consciousness**, leading to **functional impairment**.

Pathophysiology/Aetiology

- Dementia affects different areas of the brain (*Fig. 10.2.1*) depending on its cause (**reversible** or **irreversible**, see *Table 10.2.1*). **Alzheimer's disease (AD)** is the most common type (*Fig. 10.2.2*).

- In **Alzheimer's** disease there is degeneration of cholinergic neurons in the nucleus basalis of Meynert leading to a **deficiency of acetylcholine**. Other pathophysiological changes can be divided into microscopic (*Fig. 10.2.3*) and macroscopic:

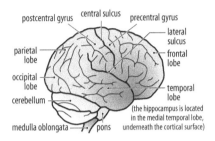

Fig. 10.2.1: Regions of the brain.

- Microscopic → **Neurofibrillary tangles** (intracellularly) and **β-amyloid plaque formation** (extracellularly).

- Macroscopic → **Cortical atrophy** (commonly hippocampal). **Widened sulci** and **enlarged ventricles**.

Table 10.2.1: Causes of dementia	
IRREVERSIBLE causes of dementia	**REVERSIBLE causes of dementia**
• **Neurodegenerative:** Alzheimer's disease, fronto-temporal dementia, Pick's disease, dementia with Lewy bodies (DLB), Parkinson's disease with dementia, Huntington's disease.	• **Neurological:** Normal pressure hydrocephalus, intracranial tumours, chronic subdural haematoma.
• **Infections:** HIV, encephalitis, syphilis, CJD.	• **Vitamin deficiencies:** B_{12}, folic acid, thiamine, nicotinic acid (pellagra).
• **Toxins:** Alcohol, barbiturates, benzodiazepines.	• **Endocrine:** Cushing's syndrome, hypothyroidism.
• **Vascular:** Vascular dementia, multi-infarct dementia, CVD.	
• **Traumatic head injury.**	

NOTE: A useful mnemonic for **reversible/preventable** causes of dementia 'DEMENTIA': **D**rugs (e.g. barbiturates), **E**yes and **E**ars (visual/hearing impairment) may be confused with dementia), **M**etabolic (Cushing's, hypothyroidism), **E**motional (depression can present as a pseudodementia), **N**utritional deficiencies/**N**ormal pressure hydrocephalus, **T**umours/**T**rauma, **I**nfections (e.g. encephalitis), **A**lcoholism/**A**therosclerosis (vascular).

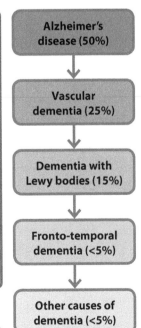

Alzheimer's disease (50%)

↓

Vascular dementia (25%)

↓

Dementia with Lewy bodies (15%)

↓

Fronto-temporal dementia (<5%)

↓

Other causes of dementia (<5%)

Fig. 10.2.2: The dementias in order of prevalence.

- **Vascular** dementia (VaD) occurs as a result of **cerebrovascular disease**, either due to stroke, multi-infarcts (multiple smaller unrecognized strokes) or chronic changes (arteriosclerosis) in the small vessels.
- In **Lewy body** dementia (DLB), there is **abnormal deposition of a protein** (Lewy body) within the neurons of the brainstem, substantia nigra and neocortex. Outside the brainstem LBs are associated with more profound cholinergic loss than in AD. Within the brainstem, they are associated with dopaminergic loss and parkinsonian-like symptoms.
- In **fronto-temporal** dementia there is specific degeneration **(atrophy)** of the **frontal** and **temporal** lobes of the brain. One type of fronto-temporal dementia is **Pick's disease**, where protein tangles (Pick's bodies) are seen histologically.
- Dementias can be divided on the basis of predominance of **cortical**, **subcortical** or **mixed** dysfunction (see *Table 10.2.2*). Cortical dementias include AD and fronto-temporal dementia. Subcortical dementias include DLB. Vascular dementia is mixed.

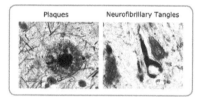

Fig. 10.2.3: Microscopic changes in brain of a patient with AD.

Table 10.2.2: Cortical vs. subcortical dementias

	Cortical	Subcortical
Memory loss	Severe	Moderate
Mood	Normal	Low
Speech and language	Early aphasia	Can be dysarthria
Personality	Indifferent	Apathetic
Coordination	Normal	Impaired
Praxis	Apraxia	Normal
Motor speed	Normal	Slow

Epidemiology and risk factors

- There are currently **800 000** people with dementia in the UK and it is estimated that there will be **over one million** by **2021**.
- Dementia increases with age (rare if <55 years; **5–10%** if **>65 years**; and **20%** if **>80 years**).
- Overall prevalence is similar in ♂ and ♀, but AD is more common in ♀, whereas vascular and mixed dementias are more common in ♂.
- See *Table 10.2.3* and *Key facts 1* for risk factors and genes associated with AD.

Table 10.2.3: Risk factors for Alzheimer's disease	
Advancing age	• The incidence of AD increases with **advancing age.**
Family history	• The lifetime risk of AD in first degree relatives of those affected is **25–50%.**
Genetics	• See *Key facts 1.*
Down's syndrome	• The mutations in **trisomy 21** are associated with the development of **pre-senile AD.**
Low IQ	• Lower educational attainment and **lower IQ** scores are associated with higher risks of developing dementia.
Cerebrovascular disease	• Strong risk factor for **vascular dementia** which can co-exist with AD.
Vascular risk factors	• E.g. Past stroke/MI, smoking, hypertension, diabetes and high cholesterol are risk factors for both AD and vascular dementia.

There are several genes which play a role in Alzheimer's disease:
- **Presenilin 1** (chromosome 14), **Presenilin 2** (chromosome 2) and **amyloid precursor protein** (chromosome 21) are genes associated with early onset AD.
- **ApoE-4** (chromosome 19) is a susceptibility gene that contributes to late onset AD. The **ApoE-2** variant is thought to be protective.

Clinical features

ICD-10 Classification of dementia

A. Evidence of the following:
   1. A **decline in memory**, which is most evident in the learning of new information, although in more severe cases, the recall of previously learned information may also be affected.
   2. A **decline in other cognitive abilities**, characterized by **deterioration in judgement** and **thinking**, such as planning and organizing, and in the general processing of information.
B. Preserved awareness of the environment for a period of time long enough to demonstrate (A).
C. A **decline in emotional control or motivation**, or a **change in social behaviour**, manifested by one of the following:
   (1) **Emotional lability**; (2) **Irritability**; (3) **Apathy**; (4) **Coarsening of social behaviour**.
D. For a confident diagnosis (A) must have been present for **at least 6 months**.

Alzheimer's disease

See *Figs. 10.2.4* and *10.2.5*.

Early stages	Disease progression	Later stages
Memory lapses, difficulty finding words, forgetting names of people/places.	Apraxia, confusion, language problems, difficulty with executive thinking.	Disorientation to time and place, wandering, apathy, incontinence, eating problems, depression, agitation.

Fig. 10.2.4: Symptomatic progression of Alzheimer's disease.

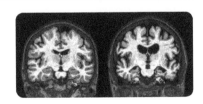

- AD can be classified into **early onset** or **pre-senile** (<65 yrs, familial) and **late onset** or **senile** (>65 yrs, sporadic), but it usually occurs after the age of 65. It has an **insidious onset** over years.

- **Loss of memory** is the commonest presenting symptom. Initially there is inability to recall new information, and remote memory (long-term memory) declines with disease progress.

Fig. 10.2.5: MRI scan showing clear evidence of hippocampal atrophy and enlarged ventricles in Alzheimer's disease (right side) compared to control subject (left side).

- **Disorientation to time and place** is closely related to memory impairment.
- **Impairment** of **cognitive** and **executive functions**:
  - **Executive functions:** Problem solving, abstract thinking, reasoning, decision making, judgement, planning, organization and processing.
  - **Visuospatial abilities:** Getting lost, impaired driving, copying figures.
  - **Language disturbances (dysphasia):** Word finding difficulties, decreased vocabulary, perseveration (uncontrollable repetition of a particular response, such as a word, phrase, or gesture), global aphasia (impairment of language, affecting the production or comprehension of speech and the ability to read or write).
  - **Apraxia:** Inability to carry out previously learned purposeful movements despite normal coordination and strength, e.g. dressing, unbuttoning shirt.
- **Agnosia:** Impaired recognition of sensory stimuli not attributed to sensory loss or language disturbance, e.g. object agnosia, auditory agnosia.
- **Non-cognitive symptoms: Perception** (hallucinations), **thought content** (delusions), **emotion** (depression, apathy), **behaviour** (wandering, aggression, restlessness).

ICD-10 Criteria for Alzheimer's disease
A. The general criteria for dementia A–D must be met.
B. No evidence for any other possible cause of dementia or systemic disorder.
Early onset Alzheimer's disease
A. General criteria for Alzheimer's met and age of onset is <65.
B. At least one of the following must be met: (1) relatively **rapid onset** and **progression;** (2) in addition to memory impairment there is **aphasia**, **agraphia** (↓ ability to communicate through writing), **alexia** (↓ ability to read), **acalculia** (↓ ability to perform mathematical tasks) or **apraxia**.
Late onset Alzheimer's disease
A. General criteria for Alzheimer's met and age of onset is >65.
B. At least one of the following must be met: (1) slow, gradual onset and progression; (2) predominance of memory impairment over intellectual impairment.

Other common types of dementia (Table 10.2.4)

Table 10.2.4: Clinical features of different types of dementia	
Vascular dementia	<ul><li>Usually presents in the **late sixties** or **early seventies**.</li><li>**Stepwise** rather than continuous deterioration, i.e. stepwise increases in severity of symptoms.</li><li>**Memory loss.**</li><li>**Emotional** (depression, apathy) and **personality changes** (earlier than memory loss).</li><li>**Confusion** is common.</li><li>**Neurological symptoms or signs** (e.g. unilateral spastic weakness of the limbs or increased tendon reflexes, an extensor plantar response or pseudobulbar palsy).</li><li>On examination there may be **focal neurology** (often upper motor neurone signs) and **signs of cardiovascular disease** elsewhere.</li></ul>

Table 10.2.4: Clinical features of different types of dementia *(continued)*

Mixed dementia	• Features of both Alzheimer's disease and vascular dementia.
Dementia with Lewy bodies (DLB)	• **Day to day fluctuations** in **cognitive performance**. • Recurrent **visual hallucinations**. • Motor signs of **parkinsonism** (tremor, rigidity, bradykinesia). • **Recurrent falls, syncope, depression.** • Severe sensitivity to neuroleptic drugs. • People with Parkinson's disease who develop dementia **after 12 months** are diagnosed as having **Parkinson's disease with dementia** as opposed to **DLB** where dementia and parkinsonian features **within 12 months** of one another.
Fronto-temporal dementia (including Pick's disease)	• Usually occurs between the ages of **50** and **60** and develops insidiously. • **Family history** is positive in 50% of cases. • Early personality changes: e.g. **disinhibition** (reduced control over one's behaviour), **apathy/restlessness** (see *Key facts 4* for frontal lobe tests). • **Worsening of social behaviour.** • **Repetitive behaviour.** • **Language problems:** e.g. difficult to find word, problems naming/ understanding words. • **Memory is preserved** in early stages whereas insight is lost early.
Huntington's disease	• **Autosomal dominant**, therefore strong family history. • **Abnormal choreiform movements** of face, hands and shoulders and **gait abnormalities**. • Dementia presents later.
Normal pressure hydrocephalus	• Average age of onset **after 70**. • Triad of **dementia** with prominent frontal lobe dysfunction, **urinary incontinence** and **gait disturbance** (wide gait).
Creutzfeldt– Jakob disease (CJD)	• Onset usually **before 65**. • **Rapid progression** with death within 2 years. • **Disintegration** of virtually all **higher cerebral functions**. • Dementia associated with **neurological signs** (pyramidal, extrapyramidal, cerebellar).

OSCE tips 1: A mnemonic for the areas of impairment in dementia (My Cat Loves Eating Pigeons)

Memory, Cognition, Language, Executive functioning, Personality.

Diagnosis and investigations

Hx **Questions to ask the patient**

- 'Do you find yourself forgetting things? Can you give some examples? When did it begin?'
- 'Do you find yourself forgetting familiar people's names?'
- 'Do you get lost more easily than you used to?', 'Are you able to handle money confidently?'
- 'Do you think being forgetful is stopping you from doing anything?'

Collateral history from informant (Also ask about functional status. See *Key facts 2*)

- 'Are they repetitive in conversation?'
- 'Has their personality changed, for example, are they more irritable or anxious?'
- 'Have you noticed any change in their behaviour, for instance being more isolated?'
- 'Are their memory problems getting in the way of their daily life?'
- 'Do you have any concerns about their safety?'

MSE		
Appearance & Behaviour	May appear unkempt with poor self-care. Behaviour may be inappropriate, e.g. in fronto-temporal dementia due to disinhibition. Uncoordinated or restless.	
Speech	Slow, confused. Difficulty finding right word. Repetitive.	
Mood	Low or normal. Disturbance of affect more common in VaD.	
Thought	May have delusions.	
Perception	Hallucinations are a core feature in DLB. May have illusions.	
Cognition	Affected in all dementias but to varying degrees depending on the type and severity of dementia. Memory impairment is most severe in cortical dementias. There is usually impaired attention and disorientation.	
Insight	May be preserved initially but is invariably lost in the latter stages of the disease.	

NOTE: MSE findings will vary depending on the type of dementia and its severity.

Ix (**NOTE:** Patients presenting with memory impairment are often referred to the **memory clinic.**)

Routine investigations

- **Blood tests: FBC** (infection, anaemia); **CRP** (infection, inflammation); **U&Es** (renal disease); **calcium** (hypercalcaemia); **LFTs** (alcoholic liver disease); **glucose** (hypoglycaemia); **vitamin B$_{12}$** and **folate** (nutritional deficiencies); **TFTs** (hypothyroidism).

Non-routine investigation (guided by clinical assessment)

1. **Urine dipstick:** Rule out UTI.

2. **Chest X-ray:** Pneumonia, lung tumour.

3. **Syphilis serology and HIV testing:** Only if there are atypical features or special risks.

4. **Brain imaging:** Imaging is only indicated for dementia if there is early onset (<60 years), sudden decline, high risk of structural pathology, focal CNS signs or symptoms (to rule out space-occupying lesions, e.g. subdural haematoma, abscess and tumour), or to monitor disease progression.
   - **CT scan:** usual imaging modality. Can identify hippocampal atrophy.
   - **MRI:** identifies posterior circulation vascular pathology with much greater sensitivity.
   - **SPECT:** rarely used in specialist centres to reliably differentiate between Alzheimer's disease, vascular dementia and fronto-temporal dementia.

5. **ECG:** If cardiovascular disease suspected.

6. **EEG:** If fronto-temporal lobe dementia or CJD is suspected, or where seizure activity is a possibility.

7. **Lumbar puncture:** If meningitis or CJD is suspected.

8. **Genetic tests:** For Huntington's disease and familial dementia.

9. **Cognitive assessment:** Folstein Mini-Mental State Examination (MMSE, see *Key facts 3*), the Abbreviated Mental Test (AMT), the Addenbrooke's Cognitive Examination (ACE), General Practitioner Assessment of Cognition (GPCOG) or the Montreal Cognitive Assessment (MOCA).

DDx
- **Normal ageing** and **mild cognitive impairment**.
- **Delirium.**
- **Trauma:** Stroke, hypoxic or traumatic brain injury.
- **Depression** (**'pseudodementia'**): Poor concentration and impaired memory are common in depression in the elderly. Identify whether the low mood or poor memory came first.
- **Late onset schizophrenia.**
- **Amnesic syndrome:** Severe disruption in memory with minimal deterioration in cognitive functioning.
- **Learning disability.**
- **Substance misuse.**
- **Drug side effects:** Opiate, benzodiazepine.

OSCE tips 2: Mini-Mental State Examination and AD

- Normal: MMSE 25–30
- **Mild:** MMSE 21–24
- **Moderate:** MMSE 10–20
- **Moderate–severe:** MMSE 10–14
- **Severe:** MMSE <10.

Key facts 2: Assessment of functional status in dementia patients

Enquire about **functional capacity** in dementia patients. The following areas of functional capacity should be explored: **dressing, continence, self-care, shopping/housework**, ability to manage **financial affairs, social contacts, safety** in the home, **ability to cook, nutrition, orientation**.

Key facts 3: The Folstein Mini-Mental State Examination (MMSE)

Generally speaking, a quick and informal cognitive assessment can be carried out by recording the following:
- Orientation in time, place, and person
- Attention and concentration, e.g. serial sevens test. Record the time taken and the number of errors
- Memory:
  - short-term memory
  - recent memory
  - remote memory
- Grasp, e.g. name the prime minister and reigning monarch

If cognitive impairment is suspected, you can carry out the Folstein Mini-Mental State Examination (MMSE). The MMSE is scored out of 30. Scores of less than 22 are indicative of significant cognitive impairment, while scores of 22 to 25 are indicative of moderate cognitive impairment. The result is invalid if the patient is delirious or has an affective disorder. Due to recent copyright restrictions only some of the items on the MMSE can be reproduced here.

Sample items from the Folstein Mini-Mental State Examination
Orientation to time
"What is the date?"

Registration
"Listen carefully. I am going to say three words. You say them back after I stop. Ready? Here they are . . .
APPLE (pause), PENNY (pause), TABLE (pause). Now repeat those words back to me." [Repeat up to five times, but score only the first trial.]

Naming
"What is this?" [Point to a pencil or pen.]

Reading
"Please read this and do what it says." [Show examinee the words on the stimulus form.]
CLOSE YOUR EYES

Key facts 4: Frontal lobe tests

- There are a number of frontal lobe tests that are useful adjuncts when considering a diagnosis of fronto-temporal dementia.
- *Verbal fluency and initiation:* Ask the patient to recall as many words as possible in one minute starting with the letter 'S'. Fewer than 10 words is abnormal. Should aim for >15.
- *Cognitive estimates:* Ask the patient to make educated guesses to questions which they are unlikely to know the specific answer to e.g. 'what is the age of the oldest person in the country?'
- *Clock drawing test:* Tests executive function. Ask the patient to draw a large clock face, put the numbers in and then make the clock show ten past five.
- *Similarities (conceptualization):* Ask in what way two objects are alike e.g. banana and orange (both fruits), table and chair (both items of furniture), tulip and rose (both types of flower).
- *Motor sequencing (Luria's 3 step test):* Tell the patient you are going to show them a series of hand movements. Demonstrate fist, edge, palm 5 times without verbal prompts and ask them to repeat.

NOTE: When talking to the patient you may register an expressive dysphasia due to involvement of Broca's area in the frontal lobe.

Management (includes NICE guidelines 2011)

General points

- After a diagnosis of dementia is made, patients are legally obliged to contact the **Driver and Vehicle Licensing Agency (DVLA)**. They may be able to continue driving subject to medical reports and annual review.
- Early discussions should take place to allow **advance planning** prior to cognition deteriorating. Topics include **advance statements or decisions**, **lasting power of attorney** and preferred place of care plans.
- In the later stages of the disease, if patients are not competent to make a decision, the requirements of the **Mental Capacity Act 2005** should be adhered to.
- **Vascular dementia** is **modifiable** and **preventable** by targeting cardiovascular risk factors.
- A summary of management strategies in AD is illustrated in *Fig. 10.2.6*.

First-line
• Supportive treatment (e.g. OT input for home safety evaluation) • Environmental control measures (e.g. motion sensors for patients at risk of wandering) • Acetylcholinesterase inhibitors

Adjuncts
• Antidepressants • Antipsychotics • Management of insomnia (e.g. trazadone) • Management of behavioural and psychological symptoms • Adding in or switching to memantine (initially 5 mg OD)

Fig. 10.2.6: Management strategies in AD.

Non-pharmacological management

- The aims of treatment are to **promote independence**, **maintain function** and **treat symptoms** including cognitive, non-cognitive (hallucinations, delusions, anxiety, marked agitation and associated aggressive behaviour), behavioural and psychological (*Fig. 10.2.7*):

- **Social support** including support groups such as Alzheimer's Society.
- **Increasing assistance with day-to-day activities**
- **Information and education**
- **Community dementia teams**
- **Home nursing and personal care**
- **Community services** such as meals-on-wheels, befriending services, day centres, respite care and care homes.
- For non-cognitive symptoms or behaviour that challenges, **aromatherapy, massage, therapeutic use of music** or **animal-assisted therapy** may be considered.

Pharmacological management

- The three **acetylcholinesterase (AChE) inhibitors (donepezil, galantamine and rivastigmine)** are recommended as options for managing **mild to moderate** Alzheimer's disease (see *Key facts 5*). They can also be used in dementia with Lewy bodies, in cases where non-cognitive symptoms cause significant distress.
- **Memantine** is an **NMDA (N-methyl-D-aspartate) receptor antagonist** and is an option for Alzheimer's disease in the following circumstances:
  - **Moderate** Alzheimer's disease in those who are **intolerant** of or have a **contraindication to AChE inhibitors**.
  - **Severe** Alzheimer's disease.
- For **behaviour that challenges**, if non-pharmacological strategies have proved ineffective, a short course of an **antipsychotic** (e.g. risperidone) can be used. For **low mood**, **antidepressants** (e.g. sertraline) can be initiated.

Principles of dementia management

- Cognitive enhancement (AChE inhibitors)
- Treat agitation
- Treat low mood and insomnia
- Functional support
- Social support
- Support for carers

Fig. 10.2.7: Principles of dementia management.

NOTE: Use of antipsychotics in dementia with Lewy bodies can cause severe adverse effects including neuroleptic sensitivity reactions or worsening of extrapyramidal features.

Key facts 5: Acetylcholinesterase inhibitors (*BNF*)

- Acetylcholinesterase inhibitors are **centrally acting agents** that work by **compensating for the depletion of acetylcholine** in the **cerebral cortex** and **hippocampus** in AD.
- They are cautioned in arrhythmias (sick sinus syndrome and other supraventricular conduction abnormalities), peptic ulcer disease and asthma/COPD. Galantamine is contraindicated in severe renal or hepatic impairment.
- Side effects include gastrointestinal disturbances, bradycardia and muscle spasms. Rivastigmine may cause extrapyramidal side effects.
- Doses: donepezil (5–10 mg OD), rivastigmine (1.5–6 mg BD), galantamine (4–12 mg BD).

Self-assessment

A 75-year-old woman is brought to the memory clinic by her children because she is becoming more forgetful. She used to pay her bills independently and enjoyed cooking but has recently received overdue notices from utility companies and found it difficult to prepare a balanced meal. She left the water running in her bathtub and flooded the bathroom. She denies anything is wrong with her when her children express their concerns. Her Mini-Mental State Examination (MMSE) score is 19/30. You suspect dementia.

1. What is the most likely type of dementia? *(1 mark)*
2. What are the microscopic and macroscopic changes in the brain with this disorder? *(4 marks)*
3. What routine blood tests should be performed on this patient? *(5 marks)*
4. What is the severity of her dementia? *(1 mark)*
5. Give six preventable causes of dementia. *(3 marks)*
6. Name four non-pharmacological management options for this patient. *(4 marks)*
7. Name two pharmacological agents for this patient. *(2 marks)*

Answers to self-assessment questions are to be found in *Appendix B.*

Chapter 11

Child psychiatry

11.1 Autism

Autism is a **pervasive developmental disorder** characterized by a **triad** of impairment in **social interaction**, impairment in **communication**, and **restricted, stereotyped interests** and **behaviours**.

Pathophysiology/Aetiology

The aetiology of autism can be divided into **prenatal**, **antenatal** and **postnatal**.

Prenatal

- **Genetics:** There is a complex polygenic relationship, with a number of chromosomes implicated, such as **chromosome 7**. There is a significantly increased risk of autism associated with genetic syndromes such as **fragile X syndrome** and **tuberous sclerosis**.
- **Parental age:** A study found that women who are **40 years old** have a **50%** greater chance of having a child with autism as compared with women aged **20–29 years**.
- **Drugs:** Babies who have been exposed to certain medications in the womb have a greater risk of developing autism. These include **sodium valproate** in particular.
- **Infection:** Prenatal viral infections (e.g. **rubella**) increase the risk of autism.

Antenatal

- **Obstetric complications** such as **hypoxia** during childbirth, ↓ **gestational age** at birth, as well as very **low birthweight** offer increased risk of autism.

Postnatal

- **Toxins** such as **lead** and **mercury** may increase the risk of autism.
- **Pesticide exposure** may affect those genetically predisposed to autism.

NOTE: There is no proven link between the MMR vaccine and the development of autism (*Medical Research Council*).

Epidemiology and risk factors (*Table 11.1.1*)

- Autism affects approximately **1.1%** of the population. The ♂ to ♀ ratio is 4:1.

Table 11.1.1: Risk factors for autism spectrum disorders	
Male	• **Males** are **4 ×** more likely to be affected than females.
Genetics/Family history	• There is an **88% concordance rate** in **monozygotic** twins, indicating a strong genetic component.
Advancing parental age	• Recent studies have suggested that **advancing parental age** is a significant risk factor for ASD.
Parental psychiatric disorders	• Evidence suggests a link between **parental psychiatric disorders** such as schizophrenia and the child having autism.
Prematurity	• Born before **35 weeks'** gestation.
Maternal medication use	• ↑ with mothers receiving sodium valproate during pregnancy.

Clinical features

- The triad of clinical features associated with autism as mentioned in ICD-10 fit the mnemonic 'ABC' (see *Table 11.1.2*).

Table 11.1.2: Autism triad

social	• Few social gestures, e.g. waving, nodding and pointing at objects. • Lack of: Eye contact (gaze avoidance), social smile, response to name, interest in others, emotional expression, sustained relationships and awareness of social rules.
Behaviour restricted	• Restricted, repetitive and stereotyped behaviour, e.g. rocking and twisting. • Upset at any change in daily routine. • May prefer the same foods, insist on the same clothes and play the same games. • Obsessively pursued interests. • Fascination with sensory aspects of environment.
Communication impaired	• Distorted and delayed speech (often the first sign which is noticed). • Echolalia (repetition of words).

- **50%** of parents have cause for concern by **12–18 months** of age. The *onset of autism is before the age of 3 years*. There is also a diagnosis of **atypical autism** after the age of 3.

- Other features include: **Intellectual disability (NOTE:** if you include all on the autistic spectrum the majority will not have an intellectual disability), **temper tantrums**, **impulsivity**, **cognitive impairment** may be present as associated conditions (see *Key facts 1*).

Key facts 1: Other conditions associated with autism

- **Epileptic seizures:** ~20% develop this.
- **Visual impairment.**
- **Hearing impairment.**
- **Infections.**
- **Pica:** Eating inedible objects.
- **Constipation.**
- **Sleep disorders.**
- **Underlying medical conditions:** PKU, fragile X, tuberous sclerosis, congenital rubella, CMV or toxoplasmosis.
- **Psychiatric:** Hyperkinetic disorder, depression, bipolar affective disorder, anxiety, psychosis, OCD, DSH.

Diagnosis and investigations

Hx
- 'Does your child ever engage in pretend play alone or with others?', 'Does your child struggle to interact with others and make friends?' **(social interaction poor)**
- 'Have you noticed any patterns in their behaviour?', 'Does your child insist on the same toys, activities or foods?', 'Have you noticed them making any abnormal movements such as flapping their hands or walking on tiptoes?' **(repetitive, stereotypical behaviour)**
- 'Do they struggle to communicate with you?', 'Have you noticed that their speech is monotonous or repetitive?' **(impaired communication)**
- 'What sort of games does your child play and with what toys?' **(unimaginative play)**
- 'Do you have any concerns about your child's development?' **(developmental history)**

ICD-10 Criteria for the diagnosis of autism

A. Presence of **abnormal** or **impaired development** *before* **the age of three**.
B. Qualitative abnormalities in **social interaction**.
C. Qualitative abnormalities in **communication**.
D. **Restrictive, repetitive and stereotyped patterns of behaviour, interests and activities.**
E. The clinical picture is not attributable to other varieties of pervasive developmental disorder.

MSE		
Appearance & Behaviour	Ritualized, stereotyped behaviour, e.g. clapping, rocking. Poor eye contact, detached. Lack of facial expression and gestures. May attach to unusual items.	
Speech	Delayed speech. Difficulty initiating and maintaining conversation. Repetitive language. May have unusual rate, rhythm and volume.	
Mood	Normal or have erratic mood changes (can appear to have a labile mood).	
Thought	Obsessions and compulsions. Intense preoccupation with special interests.	
Perception	May be very sensitive to noise, touch or smell.	
Cognition	Impaired attention but may also be able to concentrate on special interests.	
Insight	May be poor but they may be distressed if aware they are different/ don't fit in.	

Ix
- **Full developmental assessment** including family history, pregnancy, birth, medical history, developmental milestones, daily living skills and assessment of communication, social interaction and stereotyped behaviours (see *OSCE tips*).
- **Hearing tests** if required.
- **Screening tools** including **CHAT** (**CH**ecklist for **A**utism in **T**oddlers).

DDx
- **Asperger's syndrome***
- **Rett's syndrome***
- **Childhood disintegrative disorder***
- **Learning disability**
- **Deafness**
- **Childhood schizophrenia**

*See *Key facts 2*

Key facts 2: Eponymous syndromes: the pervasive developmental disorders

- **Asperger's syndrome:** Similar to autism with abnormalities in social interaction and restricted, stereotyped, repetitive interests and behaviours. However, unlike autism, there is **no impairment in language, cognition or intelligence (IQ normal)**. It is more prevalent in boys.
- **Rett's syndrome:** Severe, progressive disorder starting in early life. Results in language impairment, repetitive stereotyped hand movements, loss of fine motor skills, irregular breathing and seizures. Almost exclusively seen in girls. The MECP2 gene's role in Rett's syndrome has been identified.
- **Childhood disintegrative disorder (Heller's syndrome):** Characterized by two years of normal development followed by loss of previously learned skills (language, social and motor). Also associated with repetitive, stereotyped interests and behaviours as well as cognitive deterioration.

OSCE tips: The developmental assessment

A full developmental assessment is essential in any child with suspected autism, paying particular attention to **communication** and **social interaction**.
SPEECH and HEARING developmental milestones:
- **3 months** → turns towards sound, quietens to parent's voice.
- **6 months** → double syllables e.g. 'adah'.
- **9 months** → says 'mama' and 'dada'.
- **12 months** → knows and responds to own name.
- **12–15 months** → knows about 2–6 words, understands simple commands.
- **2 years** → combines two words.
- **3 years** → talks in short sentences (e.g. 3–5 words), asks 'what?' and 'who?' questions.
- **4 years** → asks 'when?', 'how?' and 'why?' questions.

SOCIAL BEHAVIOUR developmental milestones:
- **6 weeks** → smiles (refer at 10 weeks if not smiling).
- **6 months** → enjoys interaction.
- **1 year** → waves bye-bye.
- **2 years** → interested in other children.
- **3 years** → make believe play.
- **4 years** → plays with other children.

NOTE: Delays in language and social interaction alone indicate likely autism. Global developmental delay indicates a likely alternative pathology.

Management (includes NICE guidance 2014)

General points (Fig. 11.1.1)

- Diagnosis should be by a **specialist** and can be reliably made at **age 3**.
- **Local autism teams** (community-based **multidisciplinary teams** including paediatricians, psychiatrists, educational psychologists, speech and language therapists and occupational therapists) should ensure that all those diagnosed with autism have a **key worker** to manage and coordinate treatment.
- **CBT** can be used if the child has the verbal and cognitive ability to engage and is motivated.
- Interventions for life skills include support developing their **daily living skills**, their **coping strategies** and **enabling access to education and community facilities** such as those related to leisure and sports.
- Ensure all **physical health**, **mental health** and **behavioural issues** are addressed (Key facts 1).
- **Families** and **carers** should also be offered personal, social and emotional **support**. **Self-help groups** such as the **National Autistic Society** (NAS) are available.

- **Special schooling** may be considered.
- **Melatonin** may be considered for sleep disorders that persist despite behavioural interventions.

Interventions for the core features of autism

- **Social-communication intervention** (e.g. play-based strategies).
- *Do not use pharmacological agents* such as antipsychotics, antidepressants or exclusion diets.

Interventions for behaviour that challenges

- **Treat co-existing physical disorders** (e.g. epilepsy and constipation) and **mental health** (e.g. anxiety, depression) and **behavioural problems** (e.g. hyperkinetic disorder).
- **Modification of environmental factors** which initiate or maintain challenging behaviour, are the **first line** in management (e.g. lighting, noise, social circumstances and inadvertent reinforcement of challenging behaviour).
- **Antipsychotics** (e.g. risperidone) should be considered for behaviour that challenges, when psychosocial interventions are insufficient or if the features are severe. This requires careful consideration as there are significant side effects, and metabolic monitoring is required.

BIOLOGICAL

- Treat co-existing disorders (e.g. methylphenidate for hyperkinetic disorder).
- Antipsychotics for behaviour that challenges.
- Melatonin.

PSYCHOLOGICAL

- Psychoeducation for families or carers.
- Full assessment of the functions of behaviour, to understand the child fully.
- CBT.

SOCIAL

- Modification of environmental factors.
- Social-communication intervention.
- Self-help groups such as the National Autistic Society.
- Special schooling.

Fig. 11.1.1: Bio-psychosocial approach to management of autism.

Self-assessment

A mother presents with her 3-year-old boy following concerns about language development. He spoke his first words at 17 months but still does not combine two words. He also seems uninterested in engaging with other children. He occasionally engages with his parents but less than they think he should do, and he has difficulty maintaining eye contact. When he wants something he pulls them to where the object is and screams; he doesn't point like other children. His parents have also noticed that he does not play in the same way as other children of his age; he tends to line toys up, or plays with certain aspects of them, such as the toy car doors.

1. What is the most likely diagnosis? *(1 mark)*
2. What other questions would you like to ask in your history? *(3 marks)*
3. What is the clinical triad of this condition? *(3 marks)*
4. Name three medical conditions associated with this syndrome. *(3 marks)*
5. Name four non-pharmacological management approaches to this syndrome. *(2 marks)*

Answers to self-assessment questions are to be found in *Appendix B*.

11.2 Hyperkinetic disorder

Definition

Hyperkinetic disorder (commonly referred to as ADHD: attention deficit hyperactivity disorder) is characterized by an early onset, persistent pattern of **inattention**, **hyperactivity** and **impulsivity** that are more frequent and severe than in individuals at a comparable stage of development, and are present in more than one situation. Children may present with difficulties at **school** and at **home**.

NOTE: Adults are now also presenting, wondering whether they have hyperkinetic disorder which was not identified at school.

Pathophysiology/Aetiology

- The aetiology of hyperkinetic disorder is **multifactorial** (see *Table 11.2.1*).
- It can be divided into **genetic**, **neurochemical**, **neurodevelopmental** and **social**.

Table 11.2.1: Aetiology of hyperkinetic disorder	
Genetic	Twin and adoption studies indicate a **genetic predisposition** (concordance rate of **82%** for monozygotic twins). The *DRD4* and *DRD5* genes are thought to play a role.
Neurochemical	There are reports of a link between hyperkinetic disorder and the genes coding for the dopamine system, suggesting an abnormality in the **dopaminergic pathways**.
Neurodevelopmental	Neurodevelopmental abnormalities of the **pre-frontal cortex** are hypothesized based on symptoms of recklessness, inattention and learning difficulties.
Social	There is an association with **social deprivation** and **family conflict** as well as **parental cannabis and alcohol exposure**.

Epidemiology and risk factors (see *Table 11.2.2*)

- The prevalence of hyperkinetic disorder is estimated to be around **2.4%** of children in the UK.
- It is **three times** more common in ♂ than ♀.
- The **age of onset** is commonly between **3** and **7** years.

Table 11.2.2: Risk factors for hyperkinetic disorder	
Male	• Males are **three times** more likely to be affected than females.
Family history	• Family history is a strong determinant of hyperkinetic disorder with twin studies reporting about 70% heritability.
Environmental risk factors	• Social deprivation and family conflict as well as parental cannabis and alcohol exposure.

Clinical features (Fig. 11.2.1)

- The **three core features** of hyperkinetic disorder are **inattention**, **hyperactivity** and **impulsivity**.

ICD-10 Criteria for the diagnosis of hyperkinetic disorder

A. Demonstrable **abnormality of attention, activity and impulsivity** *at home*, for the age and developmental level of the child.
B. Demonstrable **abnormality of attention and activity** *at school or nursery* (if applicable), for the age and developmental level of the child.
C. *Directly observed* **abnormality of attention or activity.** This must be excessive for the child's age and developmental level.
D. **Does not meet criteria** for a pervasive developmental disorder, mania, depressive or anxiety disorder.
E. **Onset before** the age of **7 years**.
F. **Duration** of at least **6 months**.
G. **IQ above 50.**

Diagnosis and investigations

Hx | 'Do you find that your child…'

1. **Inattention:** '…is reluctant to engage in activities which need sustained mental effort, such as schoolwork?', '…often leaves play activities unfinished?', '…regularly loses their possessions?', '…does not listen when spoken to?'
2. **Hyperactivity:** '…is constantly fidgeting, jumping or running around?', '…is unable to remain still?', '…is difficult to engage in quiet activities?'
3. **Impulsivity:** '…cannot wait their turn when playing in groups?', '…blurts out answers to questions before the question has been completed?'

Inattention

- Not listening when spoken to.
- Highly distractible (moving from one activity to the next).
- Reluctant to engage in activities that require persistent mental effort, e.g. school work which contains careless mistakes.
- Forgetting or regularly losing belongings.

Hyperactivity

- Restlessness and fidgeting or tapping with hands or feet.
- Recklessness.
- Running and jumping around in inappropriate places.
- Difficulty engaging in quiet activities.
- Excessive talking or noisiness.

Impulsivity

- Difficulty waiting their turn.
- Interrupting others.
- Prematurely blurting out answers.
- Temper tantrums and aggression.
- Disobedient.
- Running into the street without looking.

Fig. 11.2.1: Core features of hyperkinetic disorder: 'I Happily Interrupt'.

OSCE tips: Assessment of hyperkinetic disorder

In a clinical setting, three approaches can be used to assess for hyperkinetic disorder:
1. **Observe the child:** Hyperactivity is relatively easy to elicit but be aware that a child may be overawed by the clinical context, and so any evidence of hyperactivity will be missed if the session is very brief. The child may demonstrate impulsivity by interrupting the parents or blurting out answers.
2. **Speak to the child:** Is the child able to engage in a conversation with you and do they make eye contact? Offer them a toy and see whether they get bored or are easily distracted.
3. **Speak to the parents:** Speaking to the parents will allow you to explore all three core features in more detail and to elicit whether symptoms are present in more than one environment.

MSE	Appearance & Behaviour	Fidgety. Unable to sit still. Running around, jumping or climbing inappropriately. If toys offered, will flit from one to another. If parents are asked a question, the child replies with the answer before the parents can.
	Speech	Talks loudly, even at inappropriate times and makes excessive noise.
	Mood	Normal but may be low if co-morbid depressive disorder.
	Thought	No disorders of thought.
	Perception	No hallucinations.
	Cognition	Poor attention levels. Lack of concentration.
	Insight	Poor.

Ix

NOTE: As problem behaviours vary in different settings, it is important to obtain information from teachers, as well as the parents and the child. For *adults* seeking a diagnosis, school reports are usually reviewed and a collateral history from parents is helpful.

- **Blood tests** including **TFTs** (to rule out thyroid disease).
- **Hearing tests:** Examine middle/inner ear with an otoscope and consider a pure tone audiogram.
- **Rating scales:** e.g. Conners' rating scale and the Strengths and Difficulties questionnaire.

DDx

- **Learning disability/Dyslexia**
- **Oppositional defiant disorder** (see *Key facts 1*)
- **Conduct disorder** (see *Key facts 1*)
- **Autism**

- **Sleep disorders**
- **Mood disorders** (particularly bipolar)
- **Anxiety disorder**
- **Hearing impairment**

Key facts 1: Co-morbidities including conduct disorder and oppositional defiant disorder

- **70%** of hyperkinetic disorder patients have co-morbidities including **learning difficulties** (e.g. ASD, dyslexia), **dyspraxia**, **Tourette's syndrome** and **mood/anxiety disorders**.
- **Conduct disorder** (co-exists in **50%** of hyperkinetic children) is a repetitive and severe pattern of antisocial behaviour including aggression, destruction of property, deceitfulness (or stealing) and major violations of age-appropriate social expectations. Risk factors include being male, abuse as a child, poor socioeconomic status and parental psychiatric disorders. It is the most common psychiatric disorder of childhood.
- **Oppositional defiant disorder** is defiant and disruptive behaviour against authoritative figures but is less severe than conduct disorder, in that violations of law and physical abuse of others are far less common.

Management (includes NICE guidance)

General points

- Hyperkinetic disorder is diagnosed by specialists and treatment depends on whether the patient is **pre-school**, **school-age** or **adult**, as well as the **severity** of symptoms.
- **Support** for **parents** and **teachers** is crucial. Support groups include **add+up** and **ADDISS**.
- If there is a *clear link* between food or drink consumed and behaviour, parents should be advised to keep a food diary and a referral to a dietician can be made if appropriate.

Pre-school

- **Parent-training** and **education programmes** (psychoeducation) are first-line.
- **Parent-training** is **behavioural** with parents being helped to reinforce positive behaviour and to find alternative ways of managing disruptive behaviour.
- Drug treatments are not recommended.

School-goers

- **Psychoeducation** and **CBT** (and/or **social skills training**) should be provided.
- In **severe** hyperkinetic disorder in *school-age* children, **drug treatment is first-line** with the CNS stimulant **methylphenidate** (Ritalin) being the usual choice.
- **Atomoxetine** (and if this fails, **dexamfetamine**) is the alternative when methylphenidate has been ineffective. Side effects should be monitored for.
- Side effects of CNS stimulants include headache, insomnia, loss of appetite and weight loss.
- Recent studies show no clear link between *extended* stimulant use and growth retardation.

Self-assessment

An 8-year-old boy presents to the GP with his father. The father reports that his son has recently been trying to avoid school. His teachers are starting to get frustrated as he stands up unexpectedly in class, disrupts others, seldom finishes work and shouts out answers without raising his hand. His parents report that he is uncontrollable at home and does not listen.

1. What is the most likely diagnosis? *(1 mark)*
2. What are the three core clinical features of this condition? *(3 marks)*
3. What questions would you ask the parents? *(3 marks)*
4. What is the pharmacological management in school-aged children? *(3 marks)*

Answers to self-assessment questions are to be found in *Appendix B.*

- **Learning disability (LD)** is a state of arrested or incomplete development of the mind. It is characterized by impairment of skills manifested during the developmental period, and skills that contribute to the overall level of intelligence.
- **ICD-10** divides LD into four categories depending on the severity (see *ICD-10 box*).
- A **triad** must exist to constitute a learning disability. This includes (1) **Low intellectual performance** (IQ below 70). (2) **Onset at birth** or **during early childhood**. (3) **Wide range of functional impairment** including social handicap due to reduced ability to acquire adaptive skills (activities of daily living).

ICD-10 Criteria for the diagnosis of LD

- **Mild** → IQ = **50–70** (Mental age = 9–12)
- **Moderate** → IQ = **35–49** (Mental age = 6–9)
- **Severe** → IQ = **20–34** (Mental age = 3–6)
- **Profound** → IQ = **<20** (Mental age <3 years)

Pathophysiology/Aetiology

- LD can be due to a number of different causes which are highlighted below (*Table 11.3.1*).

Table 11.3.1: Aetiology of learning disability

Genetic	Down's syndrome, fragile X syndrome, Cri du chat, Prader–Willi, neurofibromatosis, tuberous sclerosis, Angelman syndrome, homocystinuria, galactosaemia (carbohydrate), phenylketonuria (protein), Tay–Sachs disease (lipid), hydrocephaly.
Antenatal	Congenital infection (rubella, CMV, toxoplasmosis), nutritional deficiency, intoxication (alcohol, cocaine, lead), endocrine disorders (hypothyroidism, hypoparathyroidism), physical damage (injury, radiation, hypoxia), antepartum haemorrhage, pre-eclampsia.
Perinatal	Birth asphyxia, intraventricular haemorrhage, neonatal sepsis.
Neonatal	Hypoglycaemia, meningitis, neonatal infections, kernicterus.
Postnatal	Infection (e.g. meningitis, encephalitis), anoxia, metabolic (e.g. hypothyroidism, hypernatraemia), cerebral palsy.
Environmental	Neglect/non-accidental injury, malnutrition, socioeconomically deprived.
Psychiatric	Autism, Rett's syndrome.

Epidemiology and risk factors

- The prevalence of LD is **2%**: **85%** of these are **mild**, **10% moderate** and **5% severe** or **profound**.
- The ♂ to ♀ ratio is **3:2**.
- The most common risk factor is a **positive family history** of LD.

Clinical features

- The clinical features of LD vary depending on its degree (see *Table 11.3.2*) as well as if there is any underlying cause, e.g. a congenital syndrome (see *Key facts 1*).
- Common physical disorders include **motor disabilities** (e.g. ataxia, spasticity), **epilepsy**, **impaired hearing and/or vision** and **incontinence** (faecal and urinary).
- Specific causes are uncommon in mild LD whereas they are usually identifiable in severe or profound LD.

Table 11.3.2:	Clinical features of learning disability according to severity
Mild LD	Usually identified at a later age when the child starts school. They have **adequate language abilities**, **social skills** and **self-care**. There may be **difficulties in academic work**. Most **live independently** but may need some support in housing and employment.
Moderate LD	Able to communicate but **language is limited**. May need supervision for self-care but able to do simple work.
Severe LD	There is a **marked degree of motor impairment. Little or no speech** in early childhood but may eventually use simple communication. May be able to perform simple tasks under supervision. They may have associated **physical disorders**.
Profound LD	**Severe motor impairment** and **severe difficulties in communication**. Have **little or no self-care**. Frequently have **physical disorders** and require residential care.

Key facts 1: Specific congenital syndromes associated with learning disability

- **Down's syndrome:** A genetic disorder (trisomy 21) characterized by LD, dysmorphic facial features and multiple structural abnormalities. It is the commonest cause of LD.

  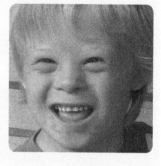

  - **Physical features** ('**PROBLEMS**'): **P**alpebral fissure (up slanting), **R**ound face, **O**ccipital + nasal flattening, **B**rushfield spots (pigmented spots on iris)/**B**rachycephaly, **L**ow-set small ears, **E**picanthic folds, **M**outh open + protruding tongue, **S**trabismus (squint)/**S**andal gap deformity/**S**ingle palmar (Simian) crease (*Fig. 11.3.1*).
  - **Medical problems:** heart defects (ventricular and atrial septal defects, ToF), hearing loss, visual disturbance (cataracts, strabismus, keratoconus),

    Fig. 11.3.1: Typical facial features of a child with Down's syndrome.

    GI problems (oesophageal/duodenal atresia, Hirschsprung's, coeliac), hypothyroidism and haematological malignancies (AML, ALL), increased incidence of Alzheimer's.
- **Fragile X syndrome:** The second most common cause of LD. A sex-linked disorder with developmental, physical and behavioural problems.
  - **Physical features:** Large, protruding ears, long face, high arched palate, flat feet, soft skin, lax joints.
  - **Medical problems:** Mitral valve prolapse.
- **Prader–Willi:** Due to a deletion of part of chromosome 15. Characterized by hypotonia and developmental delay as an infant, and obesity, hypogonadism and behavioural problems (compulsive eating, disruptive behaviour) in later years.
- **Cri du chat:** Caused by a partial deletion of chromosome 5. Those affected have a high-pitched cry like a cat. Low birth weight and feeding difficulties are also characteristic.

Diagnosis and investigations

Hx
- 'Did you have any issues during your pregnancy?', 'Were all of the antenatal scans normal?', 'Was the baby premature?', 'Were there any complications during the delivery?', 'What was the condition of the baby when he/she was born?' **(pregnancy related factors)**
- 'Is there any history of conditions, specifically learning disability, which run in the family?', 'Do you and your partner have any mutual relatives?' **(family related factors)**
- Depending on age: 'How does your child cope with daily activities?', 'Did they reach their milestones at the proper time, for instance at what age did they start walking?', 'Do they have any known medical problems?' **(clinical features)**
- Ask about associated medical problems and screen for co-morbid psychiatric problems.

MSE
- **Appearance** will vary depending on the cause of learning disability, for example the type of genetic disorder (see *Key facts 1*).
- The extent of **behaviour** problems is determined by the level of LD. In more severe cases there may be motor impairment. There is often **speech** disturbance and **mood** can be low or normal.

- **Examinations to be performed:** Cardiovascular, respiratory, neurological (cranial nerves and peripheral), weight/height/head circumference, developmental assessment.

OSCE tips: Tips for communicating with LD patients

- Always greet the patient before greeting the accompanying individual and ensure communication is clear with simple language used.
- Give appropriate time for the patient to respond.
- Use gestures or pictures to explain your point if they struggle to understand.
- **NOTE:** Focus on their abilities not their disabilities.

Key facts 2: Common psychiatric co-morbidities in LD

The following psychiatric disorders are more common in patients with learning disability: Early-onset **Alzheimer's disease, schizophrenia, anxiety** and **depressive** disorders, **autism, hyperkinetic disorder, eating disorders, personality disorders**.

Ix
- **Before birth:** Amniocentesis, chorionic villus sampling, genetic testing and karyotyping.
  - **For Down's syndrome:** Two methods, (1) Serum screening (β-hCG and pregnancy-associated plasma protein A) + nuchal translucency; (2) Quad test (β-hCG, α-fetoprotein, inhibin A, estriol).
- **After birth:**
  - **Bloods:** FBC (infection), TFTs (hypothyroidism), glucose (hypoglycaemia), serology (ToRCH infections).
  - **Brain imaging:** CT head and/or MRI.
  - **IQ** (intelligence quotient) **test**.

> **DDx** See *Table 11.3.1.*

Management (including NICE guidance)

- A **multidisciplinary approach** is vital. Care is provided by a variety of health care professionals including a **psychiatrist**, **speech and language therapist**, **specialist nurses**, **psychologist**, **occupational therapist**, **social worker** and even **teachers** (for educational support).
- The **GP** must be involved in the care of the individual as **physical health problems are common**. Treatment of co-morbid medical conditions and psychiatric problems is vital.
- **Antipsychotics** can be used for **challenging behaviour** but are overused.
- **Behavioural techniques** such as **applied behavioural analysis**, and **positive behaviour support**, as well as **CBT** can be used. Psychiatrists, mental health nurses and psychologists can support carers with these strategies.
- **Family education** is essential and support should be offered through **educational programmes** and **voluntary organizations**.
- **Prevention** can be attempted through **genetic counselling** and **antenatal diagnosis**.

Self-assessment

A couple are offered Down's screening for their unborn child. They decide against this. Eight months later after a smooth delivery, you are the doctor who performs the baby check. You note the baby is hypotonic, he has low-set ears and oblique palpebral fissures. You also observe a single palmar crease and auscultate a heart murmur. You suspect trisomy 21.

1. Give three other physical features of Down's syndrome. *(3 marks)*
2. Give five other causes of learning disability. *(5 marks)*
3. Define mild, moderate and severe LD in terms of intellectual performance. *(3 marks)*
4. Name four healthcare professionals that may be involved in patients with LD. *(4 marks)*

Answers to self-assessment questions are to be found in *Appendix B.*

Chapter 12

Management

- The basis of **psychological therapy** (or **psychotherapy**) is to help people better understand the way that they feel (*Fig. 12.1.1*).

- The aim of the therapy is to support patients in changing the way they interact with and perceive the world, to come to terms with past stressors and to cope more effectively with current and future stressors.

- Psychotherapies can be used for a variety of psychiatric illnesses, including mild to moderate **depressive illness, bipolar affective disorder, neurotic illness, schizophrenia, eating disorders** and **personality disorders**.

- Specific therapies also have a place in the management of patients with **learning disabilities, psychosexual problems, substance misuse disorders** and **chronic psychotic symptoms**.

- The most commonly used forms of psychotherapy are **cognitive behavioural therapy (CBT)** and **psychodynamic psychotherapy**. There are many other psychotherapies derived from these.

- The selection of which psychotherapy to use depends on local availability, practitioner experience, illness factors and patient choice.

- **Improving access to psychological therapies (IAPT)** is a UK initiative developed in 2006. The aim of the project was to increase the provision of evidence-based treatments (recommended by NICE) for anxiety and depression, by primary care organizations.

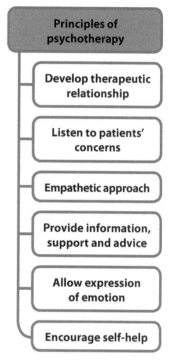

Principles of psychotherapy

Develop therapeutic relationship

Listen to patients' concerns

Empathetic approach

Provide information, support and advice

Allow expression of emotion

Encourage self-help

Fig. 12.1.1: Principles of psychotherapy.

Cognitive behavioural therapy (CBT)

- The theory/method of CBT was developed by **Aaron Beck** in the 1960s.

- Indications: Mild–moderate depressive illness, eating disorders, anxiety disorders, BPAD, substance misuse disorders, schizophrenia and other psychotic disorders as an adjunct to pharmacotherapy, as well as chronic medical conditions (such as fibromyalgia, chronic fatigue syndrome) or chronic pain.
  NOTE: CBT is an active treatment requiring patient understanding and collaboration. Patients should be motivated to participate and be able to recognize, articulate and link their thoughts and emotions.

- Rationale: Treatment is based on the idea that the disorder is not caused by life events, but by the way the patient views these events (*Fig. 12.1.2*). It is a short-term, collaborative therapy, focused on the 'here and now', the goals of which are symptom relief and the development of new skills to sustain recovery. Some people hold unhelpful core beliefs or 'silent assumptions' that they learn from early, traumatic life experiences. These people are more vulnerable to depression. When exposed to stress at a later date, these core beliefs are activated and they have **negative automatic thoughts** or **cognitive distortions** (*Fig. 12.1.3*).

- **Aim:** The aim of CBT is initially to help individuals to identify and challenge their automatic negative thoughts and then to modify any abnormal underlying core beliefs. The latter is important in reducing risk of relapse (*Fig. 12.1.2*).

- **Modes of delivery:** CBT can be delivered on an **individual** basis, in **groups**, or as **self-help** via **books** or **computer programmes** (including online). It is usually fairly brief (6–20 sessions).

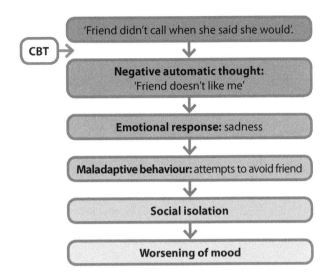

CBT

'Friend didn't call when she said she would'.

↓

Negative automatic thought: 'Friend doesn't like me'

↓

Emotional response: sadness

↓

Maladaptive behaviour: attempts to avoid friend

↓

Social isolation

↓

Worsening of mood

Fig.12.1.2: Thought process that CBT targets.

Selective abstraction

- Focusing on one minor aspect rather than the bigger picture, e.g. 'I have failed that exam because I got one question wrong.'

All or nothing thinking

- Thinking of things in all or nothing terms, e.g. 'If he doesn't see me today it means he hates me.'

Magnification/minimization

- Over- or under-estimating the importance of an event, e.g. 'He didn't talk to me at that meeting, so he must dislike me.'

Catastrophic thinking

- Anticipating the worst possible outcome of an event, e.g. 'I've got a headache. I think I have an underlying brain tumour.'

Overgeneralization

- If one thing is not going well, everything is going wrong, e.g. 'My friend didn't come to see me so she hates me.'

Arbitrary inference

- Coming to a conclusion in the absence of any evidence to support it, e.g. 'No one likes me.'

Fig. 12.1.3: Beck's cognitive distortions or thinking errors.

Behavioural therapies (Table 12.1.1)

- Behavioural therapies are based on the **learning theory**, and particularly **operant conditioning**. Operant conditioning states that behaviour is reinforced if it has positive consequences for the individual, and it prevents any negative consequences.

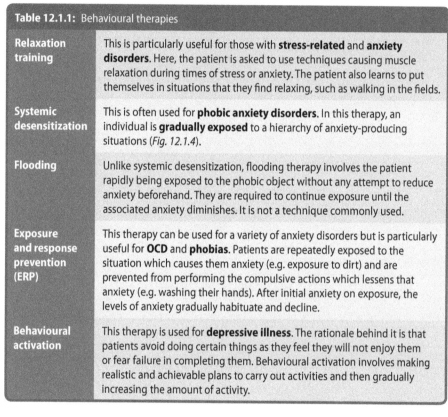

Table 12.1.1: Behavioural therapies	
Relaxation training	This is particularly useful for those with **stress-related** and **anxiety disorders**. Here, the patient is asked to use techniques causing muscle relaxation during times of stress or anxiety. The patient also learns to put themselves in situations that they find relaxing, such as walking in the fields.
Systemic desensitization	This is often used for **phobic anxiety disorders**. In this therapy, an individual is **gradually exposed** to a hierarchy of anxiety-producing situations (*Fig. 12.1.4*).
Flooding	Unlike systemic desensitization, flooding therapy involves the patient rapidly being exposed to the phobic object without any attempt to reduce anxiety beforehand. They are required to continue exposure until the associated anxiety diminishes. It is not a technique commonly used.
Exposure and response prevention (ERP)	This therapy can be used for a variety of anxiety disorders but is particularly useful for **OCD** and **phobias**. Patients are repeatedly exposed to the situation which causes them anxiety (e.g. exposure to dirt) and are prevented from performing the compulsive actions which lessens that anxiety (e.g. washing their hands). After initial anxiety on exposure, the levels of anxiety gradually habituate and decline.
Behavioural activation	This therapy is used for **depressive illness**. The rationale behind it is that patients avoid doing certain things as they feel they will not enjoy them or fear failure in completing them. Behavioural activation involves making realistic and achievable plans to carry out activities and then gradually increasing the amount of activity.

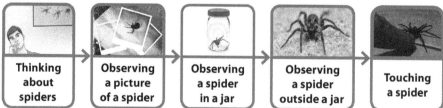

Thinking about spiders	Observing a picture of a spider	Observing a spider in a jar	Observing a spider outside a jar	Touching a spider

Fig. 12.1.4: An example of systemic desensitization.

Psychodynamic therapy

- Psychodynamic theories were developed by **Freud**, **Jung** and **Klein**.

- **Indications:** Dissociative disorders, somatoform disorders, psychosexual disorders, certain personality disorders, chronic dysthymia, recurrent depression.

- **Rationale:** It is based upon the idea that **childhood experiences, past unresolved conflicts** and **previous relationships** significantly influence an individual's current situation. It is based on psychoanalytic principles.
- **Aim:** The **unconscious** is explored using **free association** (the client says whatever comes to their mind) and the therapist then interprets these statements. Conflicts and defence mechanisms (e.g. denial, projection) are explored and the client subsequently develops insight in order to change their maladaptive behaviour.
- There is much emphasis on the relationship between the therapist and patient. Therapies can be offered on an individual, couples, group or residential community basis.
- Key therapeutic tools:
  1. **Transference:** The patient re-experiences the strong emotions from early important relationships, in their relationship with the therapist. When the current emotions are positive it is said to be positive transference and vice versa for negative emotions.
  2. **Counter-transference:** The therapist is affected by powerful emotions felt by the patient during therapy and reflects what the patient is feeling.
- **Mode of delivery:** Psychoanalysis is an intense therapy that usually involves between one and five 50-minute sessions per week, possibly for a number of years. This is a much longer duration than in CBT.

Simple forms of psychotherapy

Psychoeducation

- **Psychoeducation (PE)** is the **delivery of information** to people in order to help them **understand** and **cope** with their mental illness.
- It is usual to inform the patient of: 1) the **name and nature** of their illness; 2) likely **causes** of the illness, in their particular case; 3) what the **health services can do to help them**; and 4) what they can do to **help themselves** (self-help). PE may take place individually or in groups, and will usually take the person's own strengths and coping strategies into account.

Counselling

- Counselling is a form of **relieving distress** and is undertaken by means of active **dialogue** between the counsellor and the client. It is less technically complicated than other forms of psychotherapy and can range from sympathetic listening to active advice on problem solving.
- **Indications:** Adjustment disorder; mild depressive illness; normal and pathological grief; childhood sexual abuse; other forms of trauma (e.g. rape, postnatal depression, pregnancy loss and stillbirth); substance misuse; chronic medical conditions; and prior to decision making, e.g. genetic testing or HIV testing.
- **Rationale:** Behaviour and emotional life are shaped by **previous experience**, the **current environment**, and the **relationships** that individuals have. People have the tendency towards positive change and fulfilment which can be halted by 'life problems'. A collaborative relationship with a counsellor is one method of addressing these issues.
- **Aim:** To help the client or patient find their own solutions to problems, while being supported to do so and being guided by appropriate advice.

Supportive psychotherapy

- Is used to describe the psychological support given by mental health professionals to patients with **chronic** and **disabling mental illnesses**.

- It does not aim to produce change, but rather to **help people cope with adversity** or unsolved problems over a sustained period.
- Key elements include active **listening**, providing **reassurance**, providing **explanation** of the patient's illness, providing **guidance** and possible **solutions** to difficulties they are faced with, as well as enabling the patient to express themselves in a safe environment.

Problem-solving therapy

- Consists of a structured combination of **counselling** and **CBT**. It facilitates individuals to learn to deal actively with their life problems by selecting an option for tackling each one, trialling out solutions and reviewing their effect.
- Indications are **mild anxiety** and **depressive disorders**.

Relatively new psychotherapies

Interpersonal therapy (IPT)

- IPT is used to treat **depression** and **eating disorders**.
- The focus is on an **interpersonal problem** such as a complicated bereavement, relationship difficulties or interpersonal deficit, adopting techniques from different psychotherapies. The therapy focuses on the difficulties that arise in relationships and the impact on the individual.
- It has some overlap with CBT and psychodynamic therapy and deals with four interpersonal problems **(grief at the loss of relationships**, **role disputes within relationships**, **managing changes in relationships** and **interpersonal deficits)** which may be causing difficulty in initiating or maintaining relationships.

Eye movement desensitization and reprocessing (EMDR)

- EMDR is a psychotherapy treatment that aims to help patients **access and process traumatic memories** with the goal of emotionally resolving them.
- It is an effective treatment for **PTSD**.
- It involves the client **recalling emotionally traumatic material** while **focusing on an external stimulus**. The stimulus usually involves the therapist directing the patient's lateral eye movements by asking them to look one way and then another or follow their finger.

OSCE tips: Psychotherapy indications	
Adverse life events	PE, counselling, relaxation training.
Depression	PE, counselling, CBT, psychodynamic therapy, IPT, behavioural activation.
PTSD	PE, CBT (trauma focused), EMDR.
Schizophrenia	PE, CBT, family therapy.
Eating disorders	PE, CBT, IPT, family therapy, CAT.
Anxiety disorders	PE, CBT, behavioural therapies.
Substance misuse	PE, CBT, motivational interviewing, group therapy.
Borderline personality disorder	PE, DBT, psychodynamic therapy, CAT.

Dialectical behavioural therapy (DBT)

- DBT is used for individuals with **borderline PD**.
- The therapy adopts components of **CBT** and also provides **group skills training** to provide the individual with **alternative coping strategies** (rather than deliberate self-harm) when faced with emotional instability.

Cognitive analytic therapy (CAT)

- Combines **cognitive theories** and **psychoanalytic** approaches into an integrated therapy.
- It is based on various areas of analysis including analysing problems and difficulties, how they began and how they affect everyday life as well as analysing the reasons behind symptoms.
- Can be used for a range of psychiatric problems such as **eating** and **personality disorders**.

Format of psychotherapies

In addition to the orientation of the therapy, treatment can be offered in different formats. Therapy may be presented on an **individual**, **couple**, **family** or **group basis** (see *Table 12.1.2*).

Table 12.1.2: Different formats of psychotherapy	
Individual therapy	It is the **most common** format of psychotherapy. It involves confidential interaction between the client and provider, **permitting maximum disclosure**. The majority of evidence for practising psychotherapy involves individual therapy.
Couples therapy	Allows both partners to overcome **relationship difficulties** with the aid of the therapist. Specific issues may be addressed such as sexual relations and parenting. It is also a valuable adjuvant therapy for **psychiatric disorders** such as **depression** and **substance misuse**. Usually used when relationship problems are maintaining a psychiatric disorder.
Family therapy	Involves family members being seen together. It focuses on the family system and its ability to help both family problems and individual mental illness. Family therapy attempts to correct impaired communication and dysfunctional relationships as a means of helping the entire family including the patient with the disorder. It is particularly useful for **schizophrenia, depression, bipolar affective disorder** and **conduct disorder**.
Group therapy	Group therapy offers supportive networks for individuals who suffer from similar difficulties. Group therapy can involve cognitive, psychodynamic and supportive therapies. It is often used for **bereavement, substance misuse** and **chronic conditions**.

Introduction to antidepressants

- Antidepressants are drugs used for the treatment of **moderate** to **severe depressive episodes** and **dysthymia**.
- They are also used for a range of other conditions including severe **anxiety** and **panic attacks**, **obsessive–compulsive disorder (OCD)**, **chronic pain**, **eating disorders** and **post-traumatic stress disorder (PTSD)**.
- Antidepressants were developed in the **1950s**.
- All antidepressants work on the basis of the **monoamine hypothesis** (see *Section 3.2*, Depressive disorder) by enhancing the activity of the **monoamine neurotransmitters**, noradrenaline (NA) and serotonin (5-HT) (*Fig. 12.2.1*).
- There are almost 30 different kinds of antidepressant available today and there are seven main groups (see *Table 12.2.1*).

Table 12.2.1: Classes of antidepressants

Abbreviation	Full name
SSRI	Selective Serotonin Reuptake Inhibitor
SNRI	Serotonin and Noradrenaline Reuptake Inhibitor
TCA	Tricyclic Antidepressant
MAOI	Monoamine Oxidase Inhibitor
NARI	Noradrenaline Reuptake Inhibitor
NASSA	Noradrenaline-Serotonin Specific Antidepressant
SARI	Serotonin Antagonist and Reuptake Inhibitor

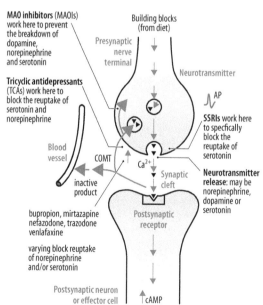

Fig. 12.2.1: The mechanism of action of SSRIs, TCAs and MAOIs.
N.B. Norepinephrine is also called noradrenaline.

OSCE tips 1: Responding too well to antidepressants!

Be wary of those patients who have an exaggerated response to antidepressants as all antidepressants can switch people with bipolar affective disorder from a depressive to a manic state. Indeed, bipolar affective disorder may be undiagnosed if the previous manic episode has not been picked up in the history or if they are yet to suffer from the manic episode.

- Evidence suggests that **SSRIs** are better tolerated, work more quickly and have a lower risk of inducing mania compared with other antidepressants. Therefore, they are generally considered **first-line** for depression (see *Table 12.2.2*).
- Research suggests that antidepressants begin to take effect by **one week** and at **4–6 weeks** the benefit is usually clinically detectable.
- SNRIs, NASSAs, NARIs and SARIs are discussed in *Table 12.2.3*.

Selective serotonin reuptake inhibitors (SSRIs) *(Table 12.2.2)*

Table 12.2.2: SSRI treatment (*NICE 2009, BNF 2015*)	
Examples	Citalopram, escitalopram, fluoxetine, paroxetine, sertraline, fluvoxamine.
Indications	**Depression** (all SSRIs), **panic disorder** (citalopram, escitalopram, paroxetine), **social phobia** (escitalopram, paroxetine), **bulimia nervosa** (fluoxetine), OCD (most SSRIs), PTSD (paroxetine, sertraline), GAD (paroxetine). **NOTE:** Fluvoxamine is not regularly prescribed as it is a cytochrome P450 enzyme inhibitor and therefore commonly interacts with other medications, potentiating their effects.
Mechanism of action	They work by inhibiting the reuptake of serotonin from the synaptic cleft into pre-synaptic neurones and therefore SSRIs **increase the concentration of serotonin** in the synaptic cleft.
Side effects (GI side effects &)	**Gastrointestinal:** nausea, dyspepsia, bloating, flatulence, diarrhoea and constipation. **S**weating, **T**remor, **R**ashes, **E**xtrapyramidal side effects (uncommon), **S**exual dysfunction, **S**omnolence, '**S**topping SSRI' symptoms (discontinuation syndrome) – GI symptoms, 'chills', insomnia, hypomania, anxiety and restlessness.
Contraindications and cautions	**Cautions:** History of mania, epilepsy, cardiac disease (sertraline is the safest), acute angle-closure glaucoma, diabetes mellitus (monitor glycaemic control after initiation), concomitant use with drugs that cause bleeding, GI bleeding (or history of GI bleeding), hepatic/renal impairment, pregnancy and breast-feeding, young adults (possible ↑ suicide risk), suicidal ideation. **Contraindications:** Mania.
Dosage	**Sertraline** (50–200 mg/day), **fluoxetine** (20–60 mg/day), **citalopram** (20–40 mg/day), **escitalopram** (10–20 mg/day), **paroxetine** (20–50 mg/day).
Route	Oral.

OSCE tips 2: Choosing the right antidepressant

There are a number of factors which influence the type of antidepressant prescribed to a patient:

1. **Overall safety profile:** Most national and local guidelines suggest SSRIs as first choice because of their safety profile in overdose as well as their effectiveness.
2. **Patient preference:** After discussing side effects of each antidepressant, it is appropriate and important to involve the patient in the decision making.
3. **Prior treatment:** If a patient has had benefit from a previously used antidepressant, that same one should be used, provided no contraindications have developed; equally if an antidepressant has already been tried and not benefited, another one should be trialled.
4. **Type and severity of depression:** SSRIs are usually indicated for all severities of depression and when there is mixed anxiety and depression. In SSRI-resistant cases, SNRIs should be tried. When insomnia is present or weight gain is desired, mirtazapine can be given.
5. **Suicidal ideation:** Avoid drugs that are toxic in overdose such as TCAs and MAOIs (see *Key facts 2*). SSRIs should still be used with caution and appropriate review (see *DO* and *DO NOT* boxes).
6. **Age and co-morbidities:** SSRIs are usually the safest in elderly. Sertraline is the safest drug post-MI. See *Table 12.2.2* for all other cautions and contraindications.
7. **Drug–drug interactions:** Avoid SSRIs in those on blood-thinning agents such as warfarin, heparin and the newer anticoagulant agents (e.g. rivaroxaban, apixaban and dabigatran), as well as NSAIDs. See *BNF* if in doubt.
8. **Pregnancy and breast feeding:** All antidepressants should be used with caution and if required, the lowest effective dose should be used. Sertraline and fluoxetine are the safest during pregnancy along with some TCAs such as amitriptyline. The SSRIs paroxetine and sertraline are most likely suitable first-line agents during breast feeding.
9. **History of mania:** All antidepressants have the potential to trigger a manic episode but SSRIs are usually the safest (avoid TCAs).

Key facts 1: Serotonin syndrome

- The **serotonin syndrome** is a **rare** but **life-threatening complication** of increased serotonin activity, usually rapidly occurring within minutes of taking the medication.
- It is most commonly caused by SSRIs but can be caused by other drugs such as TCAs and lithium.
- Clinical features include:
  1. **Cognitive effects** → headache, agitation, hypomania, confusion, hallucinations, and coma.
  2. **Autonomic effects** → shivering, sweating, hyperthermia, hypertension and tachycardia.
  3. **Somatic effects** → myoclonus (muscle twitching), hyperreflexia, and tremor.
- Management involves stopping the offending drug and supportive measures.

Table 12.2.3: Overview of SNRIs, NASSAs, NARIs and SARIs (NOTE: All of the following medications are given via the oral route)

Group	Examples and doses	Indication	Mechanism of action	Side effects	Cautions
Serotonin and noradrenaline reuptake inhibitors (SNRIs)	Venlafaxine (75 mg/day in divided doses), duloxetine (60–120 mg/day)	Second or third-line in the treatment of **depression** and **anxiety disorders**. SNRIs have a more rapid onset of action and are more effective than SSRIs (for major depression).	SNRIs work by preventing the reuptake of noradrenaline and serotonin but do not block cholinergic receptors and therefore do not have as many anti-cholinergic side effects as TCAs.	Nausea, dry mouth, headache, dizziness, sexual dysfunction, hypertension.	**Cautions** → similar to SSRIs. **Contraindications** → conditions associated with high risk of cardiac arrhythmia, uncontrolled hypertension.
Noradrenaline-serotonin specific antidepressants (NASSAs)	Mirtazapine (15–45 mg/day)	Often used second-line for **depressed patients** who would benefit from weight gain and who suffer from **insomnia** e.g. patients with co-morbid physical conditions.	Mirtazapine has a weak noradrenaline reuptake inhibiting effect, has anti-histaminergic properties and is an α1 and α2 blocker. It therefore ↑ appetite and is a sedative.	↑ Appetite, weight gain, dry mouth, postural hypotension, oedema, drowsiness, fatigue, tremor, dizziness, abnormal dreams, confusion, anxiety, insomnia, arthralgia, myalgia; less commonly syncope, mania, hallucinations, movement disorders; rarely pancreatitis, aggression, myoclonus.	Elderly, cardiac disorders, hypotension, urinary retention, susceptibility to angle-closure glaucoma, diabetes, psychoses (may aggravate psychotic symptoms), history of seizures or blood disorders, liver or renal impairment, pregnancy, breast feeding.
Noradrenaline reuptake inhibitors (NARIs)	Reboxetine (8–12 mg/day)	Second or third-line for **major depression**.	Highly specific noradrenaline reuptake inhibitor.	Nausea, dry mouth, constipation, anorexia, tachycardia, palpitations, vasodilatation, postural hypotension, headache, insomnia, dizziness, chills, impotence, urinary retention, impaired visual accommodation, sweating, hypokalaemia in the elderly.	History of cardiovascular disease and epilepsy, bipolar disorder, urinary retention, prostatic hypertrophy, pregnancy, susceptibility to angle-closure glaucoma, avoid abrupt withdrawal.
Serotonin antagonist and reuptake inhibitors (SARIs)	Trazodone (150–300 mg/day in divided doses)	**Depressive illness**, particularly where **sedation** is required. Anxiety, dementia with agitation and insomnia.	A serotonin antagonist and reuptake inhibitor.	Minimal anticholinergic side effects and relatively low cardiotoxicity compared with TCAs. May cause dizziness, sedation, gastrointestinal symptoms.	Similar to TCAs.

Selective serotonin reuptake inhibitors

DO:	DO NOT:
• Prescribe SSRIs **first-line for moderate to severe depression** unless contraindicated. • Be cautious when prescribing to children and adolescents – **fluoxetine** is the drug of choice in this age group. • Prescribe **sertraline post myocardial infarction** as there is more evidence for its safe use in this situation over other antidepressants. • Review patients after **2 weeks** of prescribing SSRIs – patients **<30 years** of age or at ↑ **risk of suicide** should be reviewed after **1 week**. • Warn patients about side effects – GI being the most common. • Counsel patients to be vigilant for ↑ **anxiety** and **agitation** after starting an SSRI.	• Co-prescribe **NSAIDs** and SSRIs, but if you have to, prescribe a **proton pump inhibitor** too. • Co-prescribe SSRIs and **heparin/ warfarin**. • Stop SSRIs suddenly – if stopping an SSRI, the dose should be gradually reduced over a **4 week period** (this is not necessary with fluoxetine). • Prescribe **citalopram or escitalopram** in congenital **long QT syndrome**, known pre-existing QT interval prolongation, or in conjunction with other medicines that prolong the QT interval, as they are associated with dose-dependent QT interval prolongation.

Serotonin and noradrenaline reuptake inhibitors (*Table 12.2.3*)

OSCE tips 3: SNRIs and cardiac disease

SNRIs should not be used in patients with cardiac disease and uncontrolled hypertension. Blood pressure measurement should be taken before starting venlafaxine and should be monitored regularly thereafter.

Tricyclic antidepressants (TCAs) (*Table 12.2.4*)

Table 12.2.4: TCA treatment (*BNF 2015*)	
Examples	Amitriptyline, clomipramine, dosulepin, doxepin, imipramine, lofepramine, nortriptyline, trimipramine.
Indications	Depressive illness, nocturnal enuresis in children, neuropathic pain (unlicensed), migraine prophylaxis (unlicensed).
Mechanism of action	TCAs work by inhibiting the reuptake of adrenaline and serotonin in the synaptic cleft. They also have affinity for cholinergic receptors and 5HT2 receptors and these contribute to side effects.
Side effects	**Anticholinergic:** dry mouth, constipation, urinary retention, blurred vision, confusion. **Cardiovascular:** arrhythmias, postural hypotension, tachycardia, syncope, sweating. **Hypersensitivity reactions:** urticarial, photosensitivity. **Psychiatric:** hypomania/mania, confusion or delirium (especially in elderly). **Metabolic:** ↑ appetite and weight gain, changes in blood glucose levels. **Endocrine:** testicular enlargement, gynaecomastia, galactorrhoea. **Neurological:** convulsions, movement disorders and dyskinesias, dysarthria, paraesthesia, taste disturbances, tinnitus. **Others:** headache, sexual dysfunction and tremor.

Table 12.2.4: TCA treatment (*BNF 2015*) *(continued)*

Contraindications and cautions	**Cautions** → cardiac disease, history of epilepsy, pregnancy, breast-feeding, elderly, hepatic impairment, thyroid disease, phaeochromocytoma, history of mania, psychoses (may aggravate psychotic symptoms), susceptibility to angle-closure glaucoma, history of urinary retention, concurrent electroconvulsive therapy; drowsiness may affect performance of skilled tasks (e.g. driving); effects of alcohol enhanced. **Contraindications** → recent myocardial infarction, arrhythmias (particularly heart block), mania, severe liver disease, agranulocytosis.
Dosage	**Amitriptyline** (50–200 mg/day), **doxepin** (30–300 mg/day, up to 100 mg as single dose), **dosulepin** (75–225 mg/day), **imipramine** (50–200mg/day, up to 100 mg as single dose), **clomipramine** (30–250 mg/day in divided doses or as a single dose at bedtime), **lofepramine** (140–210 mg/day).
Route	Oral (tablet/solution).

Monoamine oxidase inhibitors (MAOIs) (Table 12.2.5)

Table 12.2.5: MAOI treatment

Examples	• Irreversible: **Phenelzine, isocarboxide**. • Reversible: **Moclobemide**.
Indications	• Third-line for depression: atypical or treatment-resistant depression. **NOTE:** Its use is substantially limited by toxicity, interaction with food and inferior efficacy compared to SSRIs and TCAs (see *Key facts 2*). • Social phobia.
Mechanism of action	• MAOIs inactivate monoamine oxidase enzymes that oxidize the monoamine neurotransmitters dopamine, noradrenaline, serotonin (5-HT), and tyramine. • There are two main forms of MAO enzymes: MAO-A and MAO-B. Moclobemide is comparatively recent compared with the other MAOIs and binds selectively to MAO-A, therefore nullifying the need for dietary restrictions.
Side effects	**Cardiovascular** (postural hypotension, arrhythmias), **neuropsychiatric** (drowsiness/insomnia, headache), **GI** (↑ appetite, weight gain), **sexual** (anorgasmia), **hepatic** (↑ LFTs), **hypertensive reactions** with tyramine containing foods (see *Key facts 2*).
Contraindications and cautions	**Cautions** → Avoid in agitated or excited patients (or give with sedative for up to 2–3 weeks), thyrotoxicosis, hepatic impairment, in bipolar disorders (may provoke manic episodes), pregnancy and breast-feeding. **Contraindications** → acute confusional states, phaeochromocytoma.
Dosage	See *BNF*.
Route	Oral.

Key facts 2: Limited use of MAOIs!

- MAOIs also metabolize **tyramine**; therefore, eating tyramine-rich foods such as **cheese**, **pickled herring**, **liver** (of beef or chicken), **Bovril**, **Oxo**, **Marmite** and some **red wine** can cause **hypertensive crisis**. These foods should be avoided when taking MAOIs.
- Clinical features of the **hypertensive crisis: headache, palpitations, fever, convulsions** and **coma**.
- MAOIs also interact with other drugs including **insulin**, **opiates**, **SSRIs**, and **TCAs** as well as **anti-epileptics**.

Types of antipsychotics

- The first of the antipsychotics (also known as neuroleptics), **chlorpromazine**, was introduced in **1951** for anaesthetic premedication and was noted to reduce delusions and hallucinations in schizophrenia.

- A distinction is made between typical (first generation) and atypical (second generation) antipsychotics (see *Table 12.3.1*). The difference between these groups is primarily the extent to which they cause **extrapyramidal side effects** (EPSE).

- According to NICE guidelines, **atypical antipsychotics** should be used **first-line** in patients with **schizophrenia**. Indeed, the main advantage of the atypical agents is a significant reduction in extrapyramidal side effects.

- The efficacy of different antipsychotics is similar, therefore the choice of drug is often determined by the side effect profile and price. An exception is **clozapine**. Clozapine is the only antipsychotic that has been found to be superior in efficacy to other antipsychotics and is therefore indicated for **treatment-resistant schizophrenia**.

Table 12.3.1: Examples of typical (1st generation) and atypical (2nd generation) antipsychotics
TYPICAL (1st generation) antipsychotics
Haloperidol
Chlorpromazine
Flupentixol
Fluphenazine
Sulpiride
Zuclopenthixol
ATYPICAL (2nd generation) antipsychotics
Olanzapine
Risperidone
Quetiapine
Amisulpride
Aripiprazole
Clozapine

Indications for antipsychotics

- Antipsychotics are indicated for patients suffering from psychotic symptoms such as delusions and hallucinations. They are the **mainstay of treatment for schizophrenia** (*Fig. 12.3.1*).

- They can also be used for other conditions when they present with positive psychotic symptoms (e.g. delusions and hallucinations) such as **depression**, **mania**, **delusional disorders**, **acute and transient psychotic disorders**, **delirium** and **dementia**, as well as those with **violent** or **dangerously impulsive behaviour** and **psychomotor agitation**.

- Clozapine is licensed as a **third-line treatment** for schizophrenia and it is the only antipsychotic that has evidence that it is more effective than other antipsychotics.

- Clozapine should only be prescribed after *failing to respond to two other antipsychotics* (**treatment-resistant schizophrenia**).

Mechanism of action

- Antipsychotics have actions on numerous **neuro-receptors** in the brain (*Fig. 12.3.2*).

- Typical antipsychotics treat psychosis by reducing abnormal transmission of dopamine, through **blocking dopamine receptors** in the brain (*Fig. 12.3.3*). The mechanism of action of atypical antipsychotics varies, but unlike typical antipsychotics, they have a **specific dopaminergic action**, blocking the D2 receptor, and they also have **serotonergic effects**.

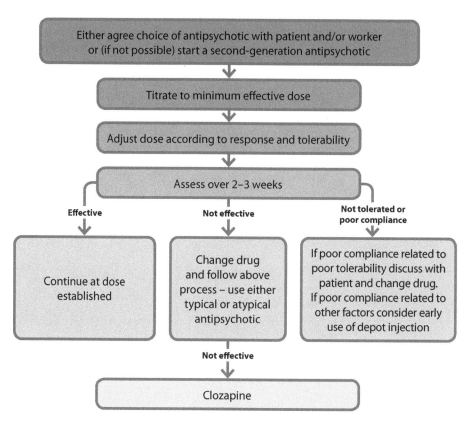

Fig. 12.3.1: Treatment of first-episode schizophrenia (adapted from *The Maudsley Prescribing Guidelines in Psychiatry*, 2015).

Anti-dopaminergic

- All antipsychotics work on **D2/D3** receptors to **reduce dopamine transmission**.
- **Typical antipsychotics** usually have a **higher affinity**.

Serotonergic

- Mostly **atypical antipsychotics**.
- Thought to improve affective and negative symptoms.
- Responsible for **metabolic side effects** (see *Mechanism of action*).

Anti-histaminergic, anti-adrenergic, anti-cholinergic

- Blocking of these receptors is responsible for many side effects (see *Mechanism of action*).

Fig. 12.3.2: The receptors that antipsychotics act upon.

- One of the main properties of antipsychotics is that they **block dopamine receptors**, in particular **D2 receptors**. However, they also have an affinity for **muscarinic**, **5HT**, **histaminergic** and **adrenergic** receptors, which explains their side effect profile:

  - **Extrapyramidal side effects** are more common in typical antipsychotics (see *Key facts 1*).

  - **Anti-muscarinic** ('can't see, can't wee, can't spit, can't s**t') – blurred vision (**can't see**), urinary retention (**can't wee**), dry mouth (**can't spit**), constipation (**can't s**t**).

  - **Anti-histaminergic:** sedation and weight gain.

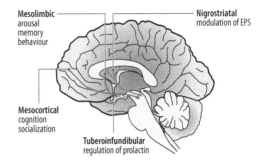

Fig. 12.3.3: Antipsychotics work on the **mesolimbic** and **mesocortical dopamine pathways** to inhibit positive and negative symptoms of schizophrenia, respectively. Antipsychotics cause EPSE via the **nigrostriatal pathway** and endocrine side effects via the **tuberoinfundibular pathway**.

  - **Anti-adrenergic:** postural hypotension, tachycardia and ejaculatory failure.

  - **Endocrine/metabolic:** ↑ **prolactin** (sexual dysfunction, reduced bone mineral density, menstrual disturbances, breast enlargement, and galactorrhoea), impaired glucose tolerance, hypercholesterolaemia.

  - **Neuroleptic malignant syndrome** (see *Key facts 2*).

  - **Prolonged QT interval:** QT interval prolongation is a particular concern with pimozide and haloperidol. There is a higher probability in any antipsychotic drug (or combination of drugs) with doses exceeding the recommended maximum. Cases of sudden death have occurred through fatal arrhythmias (e.g. torsades de pointes).

  - **Clozapine** has the specific side effects of **hypersalivation** (patients may wake up with their pillows soaking with saliva) and **agranulocytosis** requiring special monitoring (see *Table 12.3.2*).

NOTE: Typical antipsychotics are more likely to cause EPSE and hyperprolactinaemia but atypical antipsychotics are more likely to cause anti-cholinergic and metabolic side effects.

Key facts 1: Extrapyramidal side effects (**PAD-T**)

Extrapyramidal side effects (EPSE) are a major problem especially amongst typical (first generation) antipsychotics. There are four main types of EPSE:

1. **Parkinsonism:** Bradykinesia, ↑ rigidity, coarse tremor, masked facies (expressionless face), shuffling gait. This typically takes **weeks or months** to occur (*Fig. 12.3.4*).
2. **Akathisia:** Unpleasant feeling of restlessness. Occurs in the **first months** of treatment. It is managed by reducing the dose of antipsychotic and temporarily giving propranolol.
3. **Dystonia:** Acute painful contractions (spasms) of muscles in the neck, jaw and eyes (oculogyric crisis). This can occur within **days** (*Fig. 12.3.4*).
4. **Tardive dyskinesia:** Late onset **(years)** of choreoathetoid movement (abnormal, involuntary movements). May occur in 40% of patients and may be irreversible. Most commonly presents as chewing and pouting of the jaw (*Fig. 12.3.4*).

Key facts 2: Neuroleptic malignant syndrome

- **Definition:** Neuroleptic malignant syndrome is a rare but life-threatening condition seen in patients taking antipsychotic medications. It may also occur with dopaminergic drugs (such as levodopa) for Parkinson's disease, usually when the drug is suddenly stopped or the dose reduced.
- **Epidemiology:** Carries a mortality of up to 10%. It is more common in young male patients.
- **Clinical features:** Onset usually in first 10 days of treatment or after increasing dose. Presents with pyrexia, muscular rigidity, confusion, fluctuating consciousness and autonomic instability (e.g. tachycardia, fluctuating blood pressure). May have delirium.
- **Investigations:** CK (↑ creatinine kinase is usual), FBC (leucocytosis may be seen), LFTs (deranged).
- **Management:** Stop antipsychotic, monitor vital signs, IV fluids to prevent renal failure, cooling, dantrolene (muscle relaxant) may be useful in select cases, bromocriptine (a dopamine agonist) may be used, consider benzodiazepines.
- **Complications:** Pulmonary embolism, renal failure, shock.

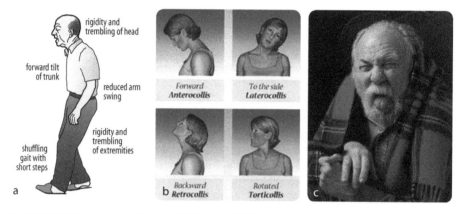

Fig. 12.3.4: (a) Parkinsonian features; (b) Dystonia; (c) Tardive dyskinesia.

Cautions and contraindications

- **Cautions:** Cardiovascular disease (an ECG may be required), Parkinson's disease (may be exacerbated by antipsychotics), epilepsy (and other conditions predisposing to seizures), depression, myasthenia gravis, prostatic hypertrophy, susceptibility to angle-closure glaucoma, severe respiratory disease, history of jaundice, blood dyscrasias (perform blood counts if unexplained infection or fever develops).
- **Contraindications:** Comatose states, CNS depression, phaeochromocytoma.

Monitoring (Table 12.3.2)

Table 12.3.2: Antipsychotic monitoring

Investigation	*BNF* advice
FBC, U&Es and LFTs	Monitoring is required at the **start** of therapy with antipsychotic drugs, and then **annually** thereafter. Amisulpride and sulpiride do not require liver function test monitoring. **Clozapine** requires differential **white blood cell** monitoring **weekly** for **18 weeks**, then **fortnightly** for up to **one year**, and then **monthly** as part of the clozapine patient monitoring service.
Fasting blood glucose	Should be measured at **baseline**, at **4–6 months**, and then **yearly**. Patients taking **clozapine** or **olanzapine** should have fasting blood glucose tested at **baseline**, after **one month's** treatment, then every **4–6 months**.
Blood lipids	Should be measured at **baseline**, at **3 months** then **yearly** to detect antipsychotic-induced changes.
ECG	**Before** initiating antipsychotic drugs, an ECG may be required, particularly if physical examination identifies cardiovascular risk factors, if there is a personal history of cardiovascular disease, or if the patient is being admitted as an inpatient. ECG monitoring is advised for **haloperidol** and mandatory for **pimozide**. Check in particular for prolonged QT interval.
Blood pressure	Monitoring is advised **before** starting therapy and frequently during dose titration of antipsychotic drugs. Amisulpride, aripiprazole and sulpiride do not affect blood pressure to the same extent as other antipsychotic drugs and so blood pressure monitoring is not mandatory for these drugs.
Prolactin	It is advisable to monitor prolactin concentration at the **start** of therapy, at **6 months**, and then yearly.
Weight	Including waist size and BMI (if possible). Should be measured at **baseline**, **frequently for 3 months** then **yearly** to detect antipsychotic-induced changes.
Physical health	Patients with schizophrenia should have physical health monitoring (including cardiovascular disease risk assessment) at least **once per year**.
Creatine phosphokinase	Baseline CK. Then measure if neuroleptic malignant syndrome is suspected.

OSCE tips: Stopping antipsychotics

- It should be recommended to patients for antipsychotics to be continued for at least 1–2 years following an episode of psychosis and some recommend continuing for 5 years to prevent relapse.
- Patients tend not to adhere to this advice and stop taking antipsychotics much before this. It is therefore essential to take appropriate measures to improve compliance.
- If stopping antipsychotics, it is important to advise patients to taper their medication over a period of approximately 3 weeks as opposed to stopping suddenly. The relapse rate in the first 6 months after abrupt withdrawal is double that seen after gradual withdrawal.

Route and dose

- The mode of administration of antipsychotics is usually **oral**.
- Some of the antipsychotics can also be given by short-acting **intramuscular (IM) injection**.
- Some antipsychotics can be given as **depot injections every 1–4 weeks** (see *Key facts 3*).
- The patient should be started on the lowest possible dose and then the dose should be titrated to the lowest dose known to be effective. Dose increases should then take place only after 1 or 2 weeks of assessment during which the patient shows poor or no response. Typical doses of 1st and 2nd generation antipsychotics are listed in *Table 12.3.3*.

Key facts 3: Depot antipsychotic drugs

- These are **long acting**, **slow release** medications given **intramuscularly** every **1–4 weeks**.
- There are numerous typical antipsychotic depots such as **flupentixol, fluphenazine, zuclopenthixol** and several atypical (**risperidone, olanzapine** and **aripiprazole**).
- Depot injections **bypass first-pass metabolism**.
- They are used to **improve adherence** with medication for patients who may find it difficult to take oral medication regularly.

Table 12.3.3: Doses for typical vs. atypical antipsychotics

Typical antipsychotics		
Name		**Route**
	Oral	**Intramuscular**
Haloperidol	2–20 mg	2–12 mg (short-acting injection). A long-acting Haldol depot is also available 50–300 mg (every 4 weeks)
Chlorpromazine	75–300 mg but up to 1 g daily may be required	IM short-acting is available but rarely used
Flupentixol	3–18 mg (18 mg max./day)	50–300 mg (every 2–4 weeks)
Fluphenazine	n/a	25 mg (every 2 weeks)

Table 12.3.3: Doses for typical vs. atypical antipsychotics *(continued)*

Sulpiride	400–800 mg (max. 800 mg in predominantly –ve symptoms; 2.4 g in predominantly +ve)	n/a
Zuclopenthixol	20–30 mg daily in divided doses, increasing to a max. of 150 mg daily	200 mg (every 2 weeks)

Atypical antipsychotics

Name	Route	
	Oral	Intramuscular
Olanzapine	5–20 mg	150–300 mg (every 2–4 weeks)
Risperidone	2–16 mg	25–50 mg (every 2 weeks)
Quetiapine	50–750 mg	n/a
Amisulpride	400 mg–1.2 g (for acute episode); 50–300 mg for predominantly –ve symptoms	n/a
Aripiprazole	10–30 mg	400 mg (monthly)
Clozapine	200–900 mg	n/a

Key facts 4: Typical antipsychotics vs. atypical antipsychotics

TYPICAL antipsychotics	*ATYPICAL antipsychotics*
Have more **extrapyramidal side effects**	Have fewer **extrapyramidal side effects**
Less **tolerability**	Overall greater **tolerability**
↓ Efficacy against **depressive** and **cognitive symptoms**	↑ Efficacy against **depressive** and **cognitive symptoms**
Metabolic syndrome less likely	**Metabolic syndrome** more likely
Weight gain less likely	**Weight gain** more likely
Less likely to cause **type 2 diabetes**	More likely to cause **type 2 diabetes**
Less likely to cause **stroke in the elderly**	More likely to cause **stroke in the elderly**
More likely to cause **tardive dyskinesia**	Less likely to cause **tardive dyskinesia**
More likely to cause **high prolactin** levels	Less likely to cause **high prolactin** levels

Antipsychotic medication

DO:	DO NOT:
• Discuss the benefit and side effect profile with each patient before starting antipsychotics. • Start the patient on the lowest possible dose and then the dose should be titrated. • Perform **ECG** and **bloods** before starting on antipsychotic (see *Table 12.3.2*). • Monitor and record the following regularly: **efficacy**, **side effects**, **adherence, physical health, nutritional status**, rationale for **continuing, changing or stopping medication**. • Consider offering **depot/long-lasting injectable** antipsychotic medication to avoid non-adherence (intentional or unintentional). • Offer **clozapine** to people who have not responded adequately to at least two different antipsychotic medications.	• Use a loading dose of antipsychotic medication. • Routinely initiate regular combined antipsychotic medication (except for short periods, e.g. when changing medication). • Prescribe antipsychotics without thought in patients with a significant cardiovascular history. • Stop antipsychotics abruptly.

Mood stabilizers

- **Mood stabilizers** are drugs that are used to **prevent depression** and **mania** in **bipolar affective disorder** and **schizoaffective disorder**.
- **Lithium** was the first to be discovered in the early 1950s.
- Other mood stabilizers were initially introduced as **anti-epileptic drugs** but later found to have therapeutic effects in patients with bipolar disorder (**sodium valproate, carbamazepine and lamotrigine**).
- **Topiramate** and **gabapentin** have been found to have beneficial effects in bipolar disorder but these are not licensed or routinely used and further evidence is required.
- **Atypical antipsychotics** have a rapid onset of action compared to the mood stabilizers and so can be used in an **acute severe manic episode** (*Fig. 12.4.1*)

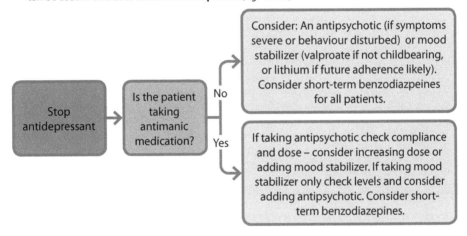

Fig. 12.4.1: Treatment of acute mania or hypomania (adapted from *The Maudsley Prescribing Guidelines in Psychiatry*, 2015).

Lithium

See *Section 3.3*, Bipolar affective disorder, and *Table 12.4.1*.

Table 12.4.1:	Lithium treatment (*NICE 2014* and *BNF 2015*)
Indications	First-line prophylaxis in **bipolar affective disorder**. Also effective in an **acute manic episode** (if an atypical antipsychotic is ineffective) and as an adjunctive treatment for **depression (to prevent antidepressant-induced hypomania)**.
Mechanism of action	Lithium is an element in the body that is handled in a similar way to sodium. There is some evidence that bipolar patients have an ↑ intracellular concentration of sodium and calcium, and that lithium can ↓ these. With lithium, a decreased activity of sodium-dependent intracellular secondary messenger systems has been shown, as well as modulation of dopamine and serotonin neurotransmitter pathways, ↓ activity of protein kinase C and ↓ turnover of arachidonic acid. Lithium may also have neuroprotective effects mediated through its effects on N-methyl-D-aspartate (NMDA).

Table 12.4.1: Lithium treatment (*NICE 2014* and *BNF 2015*) *(continued)*

Side effects (GI & 'LITHIUM')	GI disturbances, Leucocytosis, Impaired renal function, Tremor (fine)/ Teratogenic, Thirst (polydipsia), Hypothyroidism/Hair loss, Increased weight and fluid retention, Urine ↑ (polyuria), Metallic taste. *In toxicity* ('TOXIC'): Tremor (coarse), Oliguric renal failure, AtaXia, Increased reflexes, Convulsions/Coma/Consciousness ↓. **NOTE:** Normal therapeutic levels of lithium are **0.4–1.0 mmol/L**. Toxic levels are **>1.5 mmol/L** (lithium has a narrow therapeutic window).
Contraindications and cautions	Avoid in **renal failure**, **pregnancy** (teratogenic) and **breast feeding**. Caution with **QT prolongation** (including concomitant use of drugs that ↑ QT interval), **epilepsy** (↓ seizure threshold), **diuretic therapy**. Lithium is contraindicated in **untreated hypothyroidism**, **Addison's** disease and **Brugada syndrome** (heart disease with ↑ risk of sudden cardiac death).
Monitoring	• *Before lithium treatment* is started **U&Es** and **eGFR** (lithium has renal excretion and is nephrotoxic), **TFTs**, **pregnancy status** and baseline **ECG** should be checked. Drug levels should be closely monitored and patients should be informed of potential side effects and toxicity. • **Lithium levels** should be monitored **12 hours** following the first dose, then **weekly** until **therapeutic level (0.4–1.0 mmol/L)** has been stable for **4 weeks**. Once stable check every **3 months**. • **U&Es** should be checked every **6 months**. • **TFTs** should be checked every **12 months**.
Dosage	Usually given as lithium carbonate. Must be given for at least **18 months** for clear benefit. Starting dose **400 mg** at night. Titrate dose **(400–1200 mg/day)** to keep plasma levels between **0.5** and **1.0 mmol/L**.
Route	Oral.

Lithium therapy

DO:	DO NOT:
• Check **lithium levels (12 hours post dose)**, at least **every three months** and during any intercurrent illness (can ↑ causing toxicity). • At each consultation, ask about any signs of toxicity or **signs of hypothyroidism**. • Check **thyroid function, U&Es, calcium** and **creatinine** every **6–12 months**. • Inform patients: of **potential toxicity** and symptoms of this; the need for **contraceptives** in women of child bearing age; the need for **regular fluid intake**; the need for compliance in taking medication; of the dangers of crash diets; to **avoid NSAIDs**; not to exceed more than 1–2 units of alcohol per day; that it takes **3–6 months** to be established on lithium, and that **lithium cards** are available from pharmacists.	• Prescribe if you are not a specialist. • Give lithium to women of **child bearing age**. Lithium is **teratogenic** and can cause **congenital heart defects**. • Give in **severe renal failure**. • **Prescribe NSAIDs, diuretics** (particularly thiazides) or **ACE inhibitors** without careful thought. • Prescribe lithium if you feel that adherence to treatment will be a problem. • **Withdraw lithium abruptly**. Abrupt withdrawal (either because of poor compliance or rapid change in dose) can precipitate relapse. Withdraw lithium slowly over several weeks, monitoring for signs of relapse.

Key facts: Management of lithium toxicity

- Lithium toxicity is a **medical emergency** which can lead to **seizures**, **coma** and **death**.
- Lithium toxicity is enhanced by the 4 **D**'s: **D**ehydration, **D**rugs (ACE inhibitors, NSAIDs), **D**iuretics (thiazide), **D**epletion of sodium.
- If signs of toxicity are identified, lithium should be **stopped immediately**.
- A **high intake of fluid** should be provided including **intravenous sodium chloride** therapy, to stimulate **osmotic diuresis**. In the most severe cases, **renal dialysis** may be needed.

Sodium valproate (Table 12.4.2)

Table 12.4.2: Sodium valproate (valproic acid) treatment (*NICE 2014* and *BNF 2015*)

Indications	Comparable efficacy to lithium as a mood stabilizer. If lithium (and an atypical antipsychotic) is ineffective or unsuitable in acute mania. Used in combination with lithium for rapid cycling bipolar affective disorder.
Mechanism of action	Valproate is a simple branched-chain fatty acid. It is thought to inhibit the catabolism of GABA, ↓ turnover of arachidonic acid and activate extracellular signal-regulated kinase. This alters synaptic plasticity, interferes with intracellular signalling, promotes brain-derived neurotrophic factor (BDNF) expression and ↓ levels of protein kinase C.
Side effects (GI & VALPROATE)	**GI disturbances**, Very fat (↑ **weight**), **A**ggression, **L**FTs ↑, **P**latelets **low** (thrombocytopenia), **R**eversible hair loss (in 10%), **O**edema (peripheral), **A**taxia, **T**remor/**T**iredness/**T**eratogenic, **E**mesis.
Contraindications	Avoid in **pregnancy** (can cause neural tube defects in the fetus and result in **spina bifida**), **hepatic dysfunction** and **porphyria**.
Monitoring	**FBC** (to check platelets) before therapy and before any surgery. Monitor **LFTs** and **prothrombin time (PT)** before therapy and during **first 6 months. Pregnancy test** and **weight/BMI** before commencing. Check LFTs, FBC and weight again after 6 months then annually.
Dosage	Dose started at **250–500 mg** daily, and subsequently titrated upwards.
Route	Oral. IV only used for epilepsy.

Carbamazepine (Table 12.4.3)

Table 12.4.3: Carbamazepine treatment (*BNF 2015*)

Indications	Mania (**not first-line**), prophylaxis of bipolar affective disorder unresponsive to lithium. Alcohol withdrawal.
Mechanism of action	Carbamazepine blocks voltage-dependent sodium channels, and therefore inhibits repetitive neuronal firing. It ↓ glutamate release and ↓ turnover of dopamine and noradrenaline.
Side effects	**GI disturbances, dermatitis, dizziness, hyponatraemia, blood disorders** e.g. leucopenia, thrombocytopenia.

Table 12.4.3: Carbamazepine treatment (*BNF 2015*) *(continued)*

Contraindications	Caution in **cardiac disease** and **blood disorders**. Contraindicated in **AV conduction abnormalities** and **acute porphyria**. Avoid in **pregnancy** (can cause neural tube defects in the fetus). **NOTE:** Is a **potent enzyme inducer** so drugs such as COCPs will be metabolized faster. If the COCP is being used as a contraceptive, other methods should be considered.
Monitoring	Check **WCC** after a week. Measure **plasma carbamazepine levels** if signs of toxicity. **LFTs** and **U&Es** (hyponatraemia). Baseline measure of weight is desirable.
Dosage	Start at **400 mg daily** in **divided doses**. Build up (max 1.6 g/day).
Route	Oral.

OSCE tips: Mood stabilizer counselling

Mood stabilizers are dangerous drugs in that they have many side effects, can reach toxic levels and interact with numerous other drugs. A simple and effective tip for providing information on mood stabilizers is to offer your patient an **information leaflet** providing details of what to avoid, side effects and what to do if features of toxicity arise. This is a potential additional mark that the examiner will award for your communication and for aiding patient understanding.

Lamotrigine (Table 12.4.4)

Table 12.4.4: Lamotrigine treatment (*NICE 2014* and *BNF 2015*)

Indications	Used to treat bipolar depression. It is less teratogenic than the other mood stabilizers and therefore usually the drug of choice in women of child bearing age. Lamotrigine does not treat or prevent manic episodes.
Mechanism of action	Lamotrigine is thought to work by inhibition of sodium and calcium channels in presynaptic neurons and subsequent stabilization of the neuronal membrane.
Side effects	**GI disturbances**, **rash** (in around 5% of patients), **headache** and **tremor**.
Contraindications	A combination of **lamotrigine** and **carbamazepine** may cause **neurotoxicity**.
Monitoring	**LFTs**, **FBC** and **U&Es** prior to starting. Do not routinely measure plasma lamotrigine levels unless there is evidence of ineffectiveness, poor adherence or toxicity. **NOTE:** Inform patients to see doctor if signs of hypersensitivity e.g. severe rash, fever, lymphadenopathy (antiepileptic hypersensitivity syndrome).
Dosage	Must be initiated very gradually beginning at **25 mg daily**. **NOTE:** Avoid abrupt withdrawal (unless serious Stevens–Johnson rash).
Route	Oral.

NOTE: Medication side effects are commonly asked about in exams and if stuck, remember: any drug that is consumed orally always has the potential to cause GI disturbances!

- **Anxiolytics** (previously called minor tranquillizers) are any drugs that are licensed for a variety of anxiety disorders. They are called **hypnotics** if they are used to induce sleep.
- **Benzodiazepines** (BZD) used to be the main drug choice for anxiety disorders, but with increasing knowledge that these drugs cause **dependency** and **withdrawal effects**, the *first-line* drugs for anxiety disorders are **antidepressants**, notably SSRIs.
- Other drugs that can be used as anxiolytics are **barbiturates** (not used any more due to side effect profile and toxicity in overdose), **buspirone**, **beta-blockers** and **antipsychotics**.
- Hypnotics are used to improve sleep but should only be used short term.
- The following drugs can be used as hypnotics: **Benzodiazepines**, low dose **amitriptyline**, the so-called **Z** drugs: **Zopiclone**, **Zolpidem** and **Zaleplon**.

Benzodiazepines (*Table 12.5.1*)

Table 12.5.1: Benzodiazepine treatment (*BNF 2015*)	
Examples	**Long-acting** (>24 hours duration of action): diazepam, nitrazepam, chlordiazepoxide, clonazepam, flurazepam. **Short-acting** (<12 hours duration of action): lorazepam, oxazepam, temazepam, midazolam, triazolam. (Triazolam is no longer licensed in the UK.)
Indications (in psychiatry)	(1) **Insomnia** (short-term use). (2) **Anxiety disorders** including panic disorder and phobic anxiety disorder. They are indicated for short-term (2–4 weeks) relief if the anxiety disorder is severe, disabling or causing the patient unacceptable stress. (3) **Delirium tremens** and **alcohol detoxification:** Chlordiazepoxide is commonly used, starting with a dose that is high enough to control withdrawal symptoms and then reducing over approximately a week. (4) **Acute psychosis:** To augment antipsychotics for sedation. (5) **Violent behaviour:** Although they can exacerbate the situation.
Mechanism of action	BZDs enhance the effect of the **inhibitory** neurotransmitter **gamma-aminobutyric acid** (**GABA**) by increasing the **frequency** of chloride channels via the benzodiazepine-binding site of the **GABA-A receptor**. These receptors are located throughout the cortex and limbic system in the brain and function to inhibit neuronal activity.
Side effects	Drowsiness and light-headedness the next day, confusion and ataxia (especially in the elderly), amnesia, dependence; paradoxical increase in aggression, muscle weakness, respiratory depression. See *BNF* for full list of side effects.
Cautions and contraindications	Respiratory depression and hepatic impairment (where they can precipitate coma). See *BNF* for full list.
Dosage	**Diazepam:** 2–5 mg OD or BD (PO). **Lorazepam:** 1–4 mg QDS (PO, IV or IM). Max. dose 4 mg/24 hours. See *BNF* for doses of other benzodiazepines.
Route	**PO** (most common); **IM, IV** and **PR** benzodiazepine preparations are used mainly for non-compliant patients and status epilepticus.

Key facts 1: Overdose of benzodiazepines and management

- Benzodiazepines can be dangerous in overdose. Clinical features of benzodiazepine overdose include: **ataxia**, **dysarthria**, **nystagmus**, **coma**, **respiratory depression**.
- As with all emergencies, an **ABCDE** approach should be adopted and **IV flumazenil** should be given as the specific antidote for BZD poisoning.

Key facts 2: Benzodiazepine withdrawal syndrome

May develop at any time up to **3 weeks** after stopping a long-acting benzodiazepine, but may occur within a day in the case of a short-acting one. Effects include **insomnia**, **anxiety**, **loss of appetite**, **tremor**, **muscle twitching**, **sweating**, **tinnitus**, **perceptual disturbances** and **seizures** (rarely).

Other anxiolytics/hypnotics (*Table 12.5.2*)

Table 12.5.2: Anxiolytics other than BZDs	
Antidepressants	Antidepressants are licensed for a variety of anxiety disorders. **SSRIs** are first-line and are particularly useful for **OCD**. Unlike BZDs their optimal effectiveness is delayed. They are not addictive and therefore can be used long term.
Propranolol	Beta-blockers (antagonists), notably **propranolol** at a starting dose of 40 mg can be used in anxiety disorder for reducing somatic symptoms such as tachycardia, palpitations and tremor. Contraindicated in asthma, COPD, bronchospasm, heart block, marked hypotension and acute left ventricular failure.
Buspirone	Buspirone is a **non-sedating** anxiolytic that can be used for **GAD**. It works as a 5HT-1A agonist. It does not cause dependence, but its anxiolytic effect develops more slowly. Side effects include nausea, headache, light-headedness, and dizziness.
Barbiturates	Examples include **phenobarbital**, **mephobarbital**, **amobarbital sodium**. Like benzodiazepines they act on GABA-A receptors. They were used as antiepileptics as well as anxiolytic medication. Due to their side effect profile and their toxicity in overdose they have now mainly been replaced by BZDs, and are no longer used.
Pregabalin	Pregabalin does not act directly on GABA-A, but rather is an inhibitor of glutamate, noradrenaline and substance-P. It is an anticonvulsant and is licensed to be used in **GAD**, and is also used for neuropathic pain. Side effects include dizziness, drowsiness, blurred vision, diplopia, confusion and vivid dreams.
The 'Z' drugs	Include **zopiclone**, **zolpidem** and **zaleplon**. They work like BZDs by enhancing GABA transmission but are mainly used as hypnotics as they have shorter half-lives, reduced risk of tolerance and dependence and reduced psychomotor and hangover effects as compared to BZDs.
Antipsychotics	Antipsychotics are potent anxiolytics. However, their side effect profile does not make them suitable to be used as anxiolytics in their own right.

Anxiolytics and hypnotics

DO:	DO NOT:
• **Wean** patients off benzodiazepines as sudden cessation can cause benzodiazepine withdrawal syndrome. • Warn patients that hypnotics and anxiolytics may **impair judgement** and **increase reaction time**, and so affect their ability to drive or operate machinery. • Use benzodiazepines for insomnia only when it is **severe**, **disabling**, or causing the patient **extreme distress**. This should only be for a short period of time. • Warn patients that consuming alcohol can enhance sedative effects of hypnotics and sometimes cause dangerous respiratory depression.	• Use readily, as sometimes discussing feelings and providing reassurance may be enough. Consider long-term psychotherapy instead of a prescription. • Prescribe benzodiazepines **long term**. They should not be prescribed for more than **2–4 weeks**. • Use benzodiazepines to treat short-term 'mild' anxiety. • **Withdraw** anxiolytics **abruptly**. • Forget alternatives – **antidepressants** have secondary anxiolytic effects and are safer for long-term use.

12.6 Electroconvulsive therapy (ECT)

Definition

Electroconvulsive therapy (ECT) is the passage of a **small electrical current** through the brain with a view to inducing a **modified epileptic seizure** which is **therapeutic**.

Background

- ECT was developed in the **late 1930s** by Ugo **Cerletti** and Lucio **Bini**, building on earlier work by **Ladislas Meduna**.
- It was initially used **without general anaesthetic** or **muscle relaxant**.
- The mechanism of action is not fully understood. ECT affects **multiple CNS components** including hormones, neuropeptides, neurotransmitters and the blood–brain barrier.
- Evidence supporting ECT includes the **Assessment Report**[1] which analysed **90 randomized controlled trials**. This found real ECT to be more effective than placebo ECT. It also reported *no* evidence to suggest mortality is greater with ECT versus any other minor procedure with the use of general anaesthetic.

What it involves

- ECT is only performed by **psychiatrists** under controlled conditions. A thorough **pre-anaesthetic assessment** (with physical examination, blood tests, ECG and chest radiograph) is required to ensure patient safety.

- An **electric current** is applied (via **electrodes**) to the patient's skull, aiming to induce a seizure for at least **30 seconds**. (An ECT machine is shown in *Fig. 12.6.1.*)

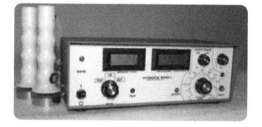

Fig. 12.6.1: ECT machine.

- The procedure occurs under **general anaesthetic**.
- A **muscle relaxant** (e.g. suxamethonium) is given by the **anaesthetist** which **limits the motor effects** of the seizure.
- One electrode can be placed on each side of the head (**bilateral** ECT) or both electrodes on the **non-dominant cerebral hemisphere** alone (**unilateral** ECT).
- **Bilateral** ECT has been shown to be **more effective** but with **more cognitive side effects**.
- Unilateral is considered if **cognitive side effects** were suffered with previous ECT, and in the **elderly**.
- Physiologically, there are **EEG changes** which are monitored (*Fig. 12.6.2*). The **pulse** and **BP** ↑ and **cerebral blood flow** ↑ **by 200%**.
- The patient usually requires around **6–12 treatment sessions**, delivered twice a week.

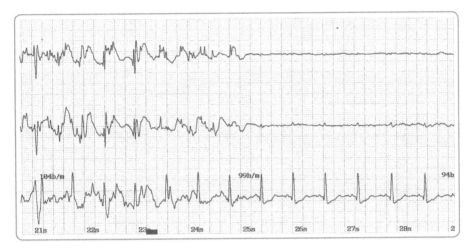

Fig. 12.6.2: EEG trace during ECT, showing initial seizure activity and termination of the seizure.

- The **seizure threshold** is the minimum electrical stimulus required to induce a seizure and it is used in calculating the electrical current dose. Several drugs affect this threshold:

  Drugs which ↑ seizure threshold: Anaesthetic drugs, anticonvulsants, benzodiazepines, barbiturates.

  Drugs which ↓ seizure threshold: Antipsychotics, antidepressants (TCAs, SSRIs, MAOIs), lithium.

Indications (*NICE*)

According to NICE, the main indications for ECT are 'ECT' (**Euphoric Catatonic Tearful**):

1. **Prolonged or severe mania** (Euphoric).

2. **Catatonia** (Catatonic).

3. **Severe depression** (Tearful):

   - Treatment-resistant depression.

   - Suicidal ideation or serious risk to others.

   - Life-threatening depression, e.g. when the patient refuses to eat or drink.

NOTE: (1) **Severe depression** is the **most common indication** for the use of ECT.

> **Key facts 1:** Consent
>
> - ECT is a procedure where **written, informed consent** is vital.
> - For patients detained under the Mental Health Act, an independent second opinion must be obtained to determine suitability for ECT.

(2) The use in schizophrenia is controversial with critics claiming that it is harmful and that it invades patient autonomy.

Side effects (Table 12.6.1)

Table 12.6.1: Side effects of ECT	
SHORT-TERM side effects ('PC DAMS')	**LONG-TERM side effects**
Peripheral nerve palsies	**Anterograde and retrograde amnesia** – the deficit is greater in those who receive bilateral ECT versus unilateral ECT.
Cardiac arrhythmias, Confusion	
Dental and **oral trauma**	
Anaesthetic risks → laryngospasm, sore throat, N+V	
Muscular aches and **headaches**	
Short-term memory impairment, Status epilepticus	

NOTE: ECT may precipitate a manic episode in patients with bipolar affective disorder.

Contraindications ('MARS')

- **MI** (<3 months ago), **Major unstable fracture**.
- **Aneurysm** (cerebral).
- **Raised ICP**, e.g. intracranial bleed, space-occupying lesion (*the only absolute contraindication*).
- **Stroke** <1 month ago, a history of **Status epilepticus**, **Severe anaesthetic risk** (e.g. severe cardiovascular or respiratory disease).

Key facts 2: ECT and mortality

The mortality rate from the use of anaesthesia is higher than from the ECT itself. The number of deaths resulting from ECT is estimated to be **1 per 10 000 patients**.

NOTE: The risks associated with ECT may be enhanced during **pregnancy**, in **older people**, and in **children**. Therefore clinicians should exercise particular caution in these groups.

[1] The School of Health and Related Research, University of Sheffield and Nuffield Institute for Health, University of Leeds, ECT for Depressive Illness, Schizophrenia, Catatonia and Mania, May 2002.

12.7 Mental health and the law (England and Wales)*

Consent and capacity

- A fundamental principle of medical care is that for treatment to be given to the patient, consent should be gained, i.e. the patient has a right to decide for themselves which treatment to undergo and which treatments to refuse.
- Consent can be **implied** (the patient does not object to, and co-operates with the procedure, e.g. sticking their arm out when approached with a blood pressure cuff) or **expressed** (verbal or written permission is explicitly asked for and recorded, often on a consent form).
- **Mental capacity** is defined as one's ability to **make decisions**. Capacity can involve consent about **personal welfare**, **healthcare** and **financial decisions**.
- Mental capacity is **time specific** and **decision specific**:
  1. *Time specific*: Person may lack capacity at one point in time but may have capacity at another point in time. If the lack of capacity is likely to be temporary, e.g. delirium, it may be possible to delay the decision until the person has recovered.
  2. *Decision specific*: May have capacity to consent for one decision but not for another (e.g. may have capacity to consent for a simple endoscopy but not for a more complex surgical procedure which poses greater risks, such as a hemicolectomy).
- The nature of psychiatric disorders means that patients may refuse treatment. Situations where treatment can take place without consent can be divided into three broad areas:
  1. Treatment under the **Mental Capacity Act**.
  2. Treatment under the **Mental Health Act**.
  3. Treatment authorized by a **court**.
- Common law is the law based on previous court rulings, which differ from laws that are created by acts of parliament such as the Mental Health Act and the Mental Capacity Act.

The Mental Capacity Act (2005)

- A person may lack capacity to make a decision for a variety of reasons, e.g. dementia, delirium, intellectual disability, neurological disorder.
- The **Mental Capacity Act (MCA)** aims to identify those people who may lack capacity to consent to or refuse treatment (see *OSCE tips 1* and *Fig. 12.7.1*) and to protect them. The MCA applies to **England and Wales** only and failures to comply with the Act are potentially criminal offences.

> **OSCE tips 1:** When to suspect a lack of capacity: **'CARD'**
>
> - **C**ognitive impairment, e.g. dementia.
> - **A**bnormal behaviour.
> - **R**efusing treatment.
> - **D**elirium.

---

*Scotland and Northern Ireland have their own laws regarding mental health, information on which can be found at: www.scionpublishing.com/psychiatry.

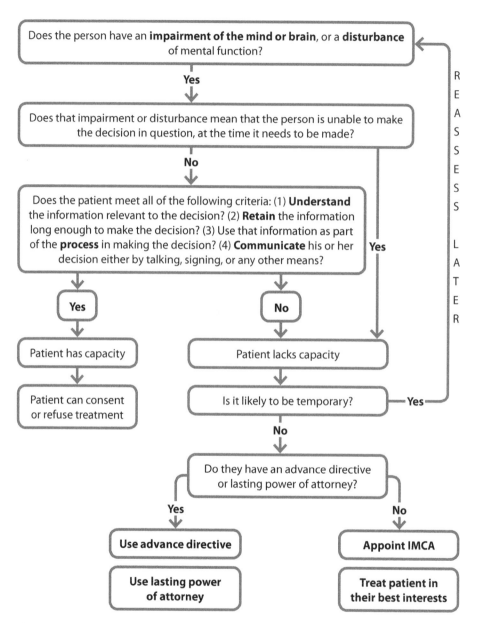

Fig. 12.7.1: Mental capacity assessment.

Key facts 1: The 5 key principles of the Mental Capacity Act (2005): 'I HELP'

1. **Best Interests:** Decisions made on behalf of the patient must be in their best interests.
2. **Help to make decisions:** People must be given all appropriate help before anyone concludes that they cannot make their own decisions, e.g. use of interpreters and multiple times (as capacity may fluctuate).
3. **Eccentric or unwise decisions are allowed:** Capacity is determined by the way in which a decision is made and not the decision itself. Therefore, it does not matter how unwise the decision is.
4. **Least restrictive intervention:** Decisions made on the patient's behalf should be the least restrictive option.
5. **Presumption of capacity:** Capacity is assumed to be present until proven otherwise.

Lasting power of attorney

- This allows a person with capacity to appoint an **attorney** (usually a relative or close friend) to make future decisions on their behalf if they lose capacity.
- There are **two types** of lasting power of attorney:
  1. **Property and affairs** deals with property and financial affairs.
  2. **Personal welfare** deals with decisions about healthcare, living conditions and location.

Advance decisions (Fig. 12.7.2)

- Advance care planning is a process that allows patients to make decisions about their future care. It takes the form of making an **advance statement** or an **advance decision** to refuse treatment, or appointing a **lasting power of attorney**.

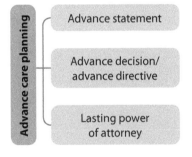

- An advance decision or advance directive is a **legal document** with a **specific refusal of treatment** in a predefined future situation (where the person would have lost capacity) that is signed by the patient and witnessed. Advance decisions permit a person to **refuse treatment but *not* demand it.** They do not allow patients to refuse basic care needs such as food and drink by mouth or basic hygiene. Persons writing an advance decision should have capacity at the point of writing it.

Fig. 12.7.2: Advance care planning.

- An advance statement (made **verbally** or **written**) allows the patients to make **general statements** about their **wishes and preferences** for the future, if they were to lose capacity.

NOTE: An advance decision only concerns refusing certain treatments. An advance statement can also be used to express other wishes and preferences not directly related to care, e.g. stating food preferences. Advance statements are **not legally binding** like advance decisions.

Deprivation of Liberty Safeguard (DoLS)

- The aim of **DoLS** is to make sure that people in care homes, hospitals and supported living, who **lack capacity**, are looked after in a way that **does not inappropriately restrict their freedom**.
- When a hospital or care home identifies that a person who lacks capacity is being, or risks being deprived of their liberty, they must apply for an authorization of deprivation of liberty.

Independent Mental Capacity Advocate (IMCA)

- An **IMCA** is someone appointed to support a person who lacks capacity but has no one to speak on their behalf (i.e. no next of kin or lasting power of attorney).
- The IMCA makes representations about the person's wishes, feelings, beliefs and values, while bringing to the attention of the decision maker all factors that are relevant to the decision.

The Mental Health Act (1983, amended in 2007)

Introduction

- The **Mental Health Act (MHA)** (1983, amended in 2007) is the law in **England and Wales** that allows people with a '**mental disorder**' (see *Key facts 2* for definition) to be **sectioned**, i.e. **admitted** to hospital, **detained** and **treated without their consent** – either for their **own health and safety**, or for the **protection of other people**.
- This is used for individuals who will **not** consent to be admitted voluntarily, or who lack capacity to consent to admission and treatment.

> **Key facts 2:** Definition of a mental disorder
>
> A mental disorder is defined as any **disorder** or **disability** of the **mind**. It includes **mental illness, personality disorder, learning disability** and **disorders of sexual preference** (e.g. paedophilia), but **NOT** dependence on **alcohol** or **drugs**.

- Patients who are only under the **influence of alcohol** or **drugs** are **specifically excluded**.
- Scotland and Northern Ireland have their own laws, information on which can be found at www.scionpublishing.com/psychiatry.
- People can fit under different sections of the Mental Health Act, depending on the circumstances (*Fig. 12.7.3*). People who are compulsorily admitted to hospital are called '**formal**' or '**involuntary**' patients.
- **Sections 2** and **3** are the **most common** sections of the MHA that are used to admit people.
- See *Table 12.7.1* for common abbreviations related to the MHA.

Table 12.7.1: Common abbreviations related to the Mental Health Act (MHA)

- **MHAC: Mental Health Act Commission** (MHA is supervised by this commission).
- **AMHP: Approved mental health professional** (they make an application for the patient to be sectioned. They may be social workers, nurses, psychologists or OTs, but not doctors).
- **AC: Approved clinician** (almost always doctors but can be other professionals. If they are section 12, it means they are approved by the Secretary of State as having expertise in the assessment and treatment of mental disorders as described in Section 12 of the MHA).
- **NR: Nearest relative.**
- **CTO: Community treatment order** (see *CTO subsection*).

OSCE tips 2: When to use the Mental Health Act (1983/2007) - '**Revise Our Mental Health Act**'

- **R**efusal of voluntary treatment.
- **O**ther options have been considered but are not appropriate.
- **M**ental disorder: The behaviour must be the result of a known or suspected mental disorder.
- **H**arm (risk of): The person must be at significant risk of self-harm, self-neglect or harm to others.
- **A**ppropriate treatment: There must be an appropriate treatment option available to the patient.

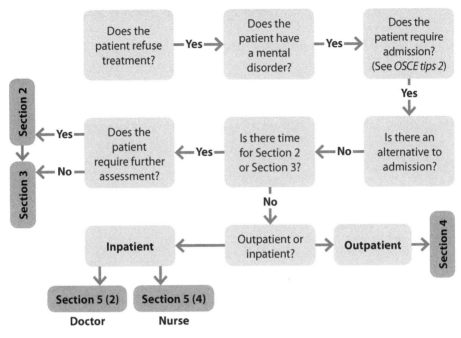

Fig. 12.7.3: Deciding when to use the MHA.

Sections 2 and 3

- **Purpose: Section 2 (s2)** allows for an admission, for **assessment** and **response** to treatment. It lasts up to **28 days**. The purpose of **section 3 (s3)** is for the **treatment** of a mental disorder. Patients can be detained under s3 if they are well known to mental health services or following an admission under s2. For s3, patients can be detained for up to **6 months**, but may be discharged before this. Detention under s3 can be renewed for a further 6 months. After that, detention can be renewed for further periods of one year at a time.

- **Recommendations:** For s2 and 3, an **AMHP** or rarely the **NR** makes the application on the **recommendation of two approved clinicians** with at least one **section 12** approved doctor.

- **Patient's rights:**

  - A patient under s2 can appeal against the section to a **tribunal** during the **first 14 days** and to **hospital managers** at any time.

  - **For s3**, patients have the right to appeal against detention to a tribunal (only **one time**) during the **first 6 months** of detention. If the s3 is renewed, an appeal can be made **once** during the **second 6 months**. Then an appeal can be made once during each one-year period.

  - Patients have the right to apply for discharge to the **Mental Health Act managers** at any time whilst they are detained and an **Independent Mental Health Advocate** can be sought to raise any issues patients have with their care and treatment.

  - Under s2 and s3, patients can't refuse treatment. Under s3, patients can be treated against their will for **3 months**, but after this time they are seen by a **second opinion appointed doctor (SOAD)** if they lack capacity to consent or are refusing treatment. A SOAD carries out an assessment to see if they think that the treatment is needed.

- Some treatments can't be given without consent unless certain criteria are met. These treatments include **ECT**.
- Aftercare: Free aftercare is provided for patients when discharged from s3. This is known as **section 117 aftercare**.

The emergency sections

All last up to **72 hours** apart from section 5(4) which is up to 6 hours:

- Section 4: Used as an **emergency**, when **s2** would involve an **unacceptable delay**. Often changed to a section 2 upon arrival at hospital. It can be done by **one doctor** with an **AMHP** or **nearest relative (NR)**. There is **no right to appeal**.
- Section 5 (2): Is the urgent detention of **inpatients** on any ward excluding A&E, by an AC. Patients on **s5(2)** must then be assessed for s2 or s3 or discharge from s5(2) to become an informal patient. There is **no right to appeal**.
- Section 5 (4): Allows urgent detention for up to **6 hours** of an **inpatient** already receiving treatment for a mental disorder in hospital. It is carried out by a **registered mental health nurse** when a doctor is unable to attend immediately. There is **no right to appeal**.
- Section 135: Allows a **police officer** or authorized person with a **magistrate's warrant** to enter a person's **premises**, who is suspected of suffering from a mental disorder, and remove them to a place of safety.
- Section 136: Allows a **police officer** to remove an individual, who appears to suffer from a mental disorder, from a **public place** to a place of safety for assessment.

Community treatment order

- A **community treatment order (CTO)** allows patients on s3 who are well enough, to leave the hospital for treatment in the community.
- The decision is made by the responsible clinician (RC) with the agreement of the AMHP.
- The patient can be recalled to hospital if they do not comply with treatment or attend appointments. Once recalled they may be detained for up to 72 hours for assessment.

Other notable sections

- Section 117: Deals with aftercare responsibilities after a patient has been detained under s3.
- Sections 35–38: Used by a court to send offenders to hospital for psychiatric assessment.
- Section 7 (guardianship): Gives power to specify where the patient lives and requires them to give professionals involved in their care, access to their home.
- Sections 58 and 59: Deal with treatments requiring consent *or* second opinion and consent *and* second opinion, respectively.
- Section 62: Concerns urgent treatments such as ECT for life-threatening depression.
- See *Key facts 3* for a summary of main civil sections that are likely to be tested in exams.

Key facts 3: Summary of main civil sections

Section	Purpose	Order	Who can enforce?	Duration
2	Admission for *assessment* – **not renewable**.	Assessment	An AMHP or rarely the NR makes the application on the recommendation of two doctors. One of the doctors should be 'approved' under Section 12 of the MHA (usually a consultant psychiatrist).	28 days
3	Admission for *treatment* – **renewable**.	Treatment	Same as above.	6 months
4	Used as an emergency, when a section 2 would involve an unacceptable delay. Often changed to a section 2 upon arrival at hospital.	Emergency	GP and AMHP or NR.	72 hours
5 (2)	A patient who is a voluntary patient in hospital can be legally detained by a doctor.	Holding	Doctor.	72 hours
5 (4)	Similar to section 5(2) but completed by nursing staff.	Holding	Nurse.	6 hours
135	A court order can be obtained to allow the police to break into a property to remove a person to a place of safety.	Police	Magistrate/Police officer.	72 hours
136	Someone found in a public place who appears to have a mental disorder can be taken by the police to a place of safety.	Police	Police officer.	72 hours

Chapter 13

Forensic psychiatry

What is forensic psychiatry?

- **Forensic psychiatry** is a branch of psychiatry that deals with the **assessment and treatment** of **mentally disordered offenders**. It deals with the interface between psychiatry and the criminal justice system.
- There is a significantly **higher prevalence** of mental illness among **prisoners** as compared to the general population. More than **70%** of prisoners have a mental disorder.
- The **1983 Mental Health Act** of England and Wales has specific **forensic sections** for patients in prison, or those who are being directed to hospital from court.
- Forensic mental health services may support a patient:
  - Who was unwell at the time of committing the offence.
  - In prison for an offence unrelated to a mental health problem, who becomes unwell whilst in prison.
  - With mental health problems in the community who has a significant history of risk issues or poses significant risk to others.
- The forensic psychiatrist has many roles which include:
  - Psychiatric assessment (and if appropriate, treatment and rehabilitation) of offenders charged with a serious crime.
  - Providing treatment for convicted prisoners charged with a serious crime.
  - Assessment and treatment of non-offenders with difficult or dangerous behaviour in a secure setting (see *Table 13.1*).
  - Giving advice to other psychiatrists encountering forensic issues.
- See *Fig. 13.1* and *Key facts 2* for specific psychiatric conditions associated with crime.

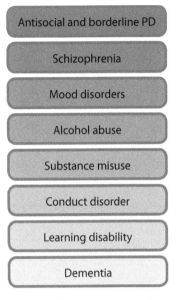

Antisocial and borderline PD

Schizophrenia

Mood disorders

Alcohol abuse

Substance misuse

Conduct disorder

Learning disability

Dementia

Fig. 13.1: Conditions associated with crime.

Table 13.1: Psychiatric inpatient settings	
Setting	**Description**
Open ward	Admission wards in local psychiatric hospitals.
Low secure	Definition is not as clear as medium and high secure. Less physical security than medium secure units but more than standard open psychiatric wards. Have locked doors. Often transferred here if other mental health services cannot treat you due to challenging behaviour and/or risk to others.
Medium secure	Not as secure as high secure services. Have air locked entrances, unbreakable windows, and high nurse to patient ratios, with restraint training for staff.
High secure	For those who present an immediate and grave danger to the general public because they are violent, unstable or dangerous. There are three units in England: Ashworth (Merseyside), Broadmoor (Berkshire) and Rampton (Nottinghamshire).

Court proceedings

- There are two main considerations in court proceedings. These are **fitness to plead** and **criminal responsibility** (see *Key facts 1*).
- Fitness to plead is the capacity for an offender to mount a defence against his or her charges. A jury determines whether the charged can:
  - **Understand the nature of the charges** and the meaning of guilty and non-guilty pleas.
  - **Challenge jurors.**
  - **Instruct a solicitor.**
  - **Follow court proceedings** and the evidence presented before the court.

Key facts 1: *Mens rea* (guilty mind)

It should be determined whether the convicted understood the nature of the unlawful act and what their intentions were. If they fully intended to commit the act and were aware of the ramifications, this is known as *mens rea*. There are a number of circumstances in which a defendant may lack *mens rea*:

- **Age:** By default, children under the age of 10 are deemed incapable of criminal intent. Those between the ages of 10 and 14 are not criminally responsible unless the prosecution can prove otherwise. After the age of 14, individuals are legally responsible for their actions.
- **Diminished responsibility:** Only applies in relation to charges of murder. If successful the charge of murder will be changed to a charge of manslaughter which has more flexible sentencing. The defendant must have an 'abnormality of mind' as defined in the Homicide Act (1957). This defence could be used if a patient with schizophrenia commits a murder as a direct result of his/her mental health problems.
- **Automatism:** An act committed without presence of mind (e.g. during sleepwalking).

Predictors of violent behaviour

Risk factors for violence can be divided into demographic and personal (see *Table 13.2*).

Table 13.2: Risk factors for violence

Demographic	Personal
• Male. • Young age. • Low socioeconomic status. • Lack of social support (lack of friends, marital issues). • Access to weapons or other means of violence.	• Past history of violent behaviour. • Substance misuse and alcohol abuse. • Major psychiatric illness (*Fig. 13.1*). • Difficult upbringing, e.g. childhood abuse and parental fighting. • Impulsivity.

Key facts 2: Specific associations between a psychiatric condition and the offence

- **Depression:** Shoplifting, homicide and infanticide (in postnatal depression).
- **Mania:** Violence (usually minor), reckless driving, inappropriate sexual behaviour.
- **Schizophrenia** and **personality disorder:** Violent acts (e.g. assault, murder).
- **Learning disability:** Sexual offences, arson.
- **Dementia:** Shoplifting, violence, inappropriate sexual behaviour (e.g. indecent exposure).
- **Alcohol** and **substance misuse:** Violence (assault), driving offences.

OSCE tips: Features to look out for in the MSE that may indicate impending violence

- Expressed violent intentions or direct threats.
- Paranoid delusions, delusions of control or morbid jealousy.
- Second person auditory (command) hallucinations encouraging patient to commit violent act.
- Disinhibited behaviour or irritable mood.

Chapter 14

Common OSCE scenarios and mark schemes

This section is most suited for group study in the weeks leading up to your OSCE examinations. The section includes:

1. **Student briefing:** Contains the candidate instructions and time allowance.
2. **Simulated patient briefing:** Includes the directions and instructions for the simulated patient.
3. **Mark schemes:** This contains a checklist of tasks and competencies which the candidate is expected to complete within the station. There are also a number of potential questions which an examiner may have for a candidate.

These scenarios and mark schemes will vary between universities and these should be used to aid your revision. You will need to familiarize yourself with the examination structure within your own institution.

Student briefing

Station 1

You are a junior doctor working in General Practice. Mrs Cook has come to see you because she has been feeling very tired and low in mood. Please take a history. You have 10 minutes.

Station 2

You are a junior doctor in A&E. A 24-year-old man has been brought in by his family because he has been acting 'very strangely' and they are very concerned about his recent behaviour. Please take a history and perform a mental state examination. You have 20 minutes.

Station 3

You are a junior doctor in A&E. The police have brought in a 30-year-old woman who was found playing guitar in the middle of the night in her next door neighbour's garden. Please take a history and perform a mental state examination. You have 20 minutes.

Station 4

You are a junior doctor in A&E. You have come to see Miss West who has been brought in by her partner because she took an overdose of paracetamol following an argument. She is now medically stabilized. Please take a psychiatric history focusing particularly on the risk, in order to be able to make a clear management plan. You have 10 minutes.

Station 5

You are a junior doctor working in General Practice. Mr Anderson has been brought in by his wife because she believes his drinking has become out of control. Please take a history from Mr Anderson. You have 10 minutes.

Simulated patient briefing

Station 1

Patient's details

Patient's name: Sandra Cook

Patient's age: 37 years

Patient's occupation: Unemployed

Presenting complaint

- You have come to see your GP because you have been feeling very tired and low in mood. This has been going on for 3 months.
- You find it difficult to fall asleep and strangely wake up earlier in the morning than usual and are then unable to fall asleep again. You used to wake at 7am, and now find yourself wide awake at 4am, despite feeling extremely tired all of the time. You do not sleep during the day.
- You also lack enjoyment in the things you used to enjoy, which was going out with friends and going for walks.
- All of these symptoms started to develop when you lost your job as a financial advisor, 4 months ago. You are currently unemployed and are on Jobseeker's Allowance.
- You have also found that your relationship with your husband has diminished as he feels frustrated by your lack of interest in everything, including having sex.
- You have lost your appetite and have noticed that your clothes have become looser, although you haven't measured your weight recently.
- You feel worthless as a mother and as a wife, and feel guilty for the way that you feel.
- You have no thoughts of self-harm or suicide as you would never put your two children through that.
- You do not have any psychotic symptoms.
- There is no past history of any psychiatric or mental health conditions.

Past medical history and drug history

No medical history of note. No regular medication, and you have never used illicit drugs. NKDA.

Social history

- You do not smoke or drink alcohol and have never taken any illicit drugs.
- You live at home with your husband and two children.

Ideas, concerns and expectations

- You know that a problem exists but are not sure what it could be.
- You are concerned that the children are also suffering because you think you are an unfit mother.
- You are hoping for some form of counselling.

Diagnosis

Moderate to severe depression.

Differentials

- Other depressive disorders e.g. dysthymia, seasonal affective disorder.
- Bipolar affective disorder.
- Organic disorder, e.g. hypothyroidism.

Station 2

Patient's details

Patient's name: Jermaine Powell

Patient age: 24 years

Patient's occupation: Restaurant waiter

Presenting complaint

- When asked why you are here you are not sure and say that you are fine.
- You appear slightly restless and appear to be responding to voices that are talking about you.
- You can hear voices that are commenting on what you are doing. There are two voices which you do not recognize. This has been very distressing for you. The voices are not talking directly to you. The voices started when you were at home only, but now you hear them wherever you go. You can hear them in the hospital. You do not understand how this is happening.
- For approximately 2 weeks, you feel that the police and FBI are after you because you have access to top secret information. They are trying to access your thoughts and you sometimes feel that your thoughts are not your own. You are very defensive if questioned about whether this is actually true because your family and friends have not believed you and you are already very upset about this and do not trust anyone.
- You are in control of your actions, thoughts and behaviours (passivity phenomenon) if asked about this.
- You do not have any formal thought disorder or disorders of speech.
- You do not feel depressed and you are not elated in mood.

Ideas, concerns and expectations

You have no insight that you could be suffering from a mental disorder. You are concerned that the police and FBI will torture you. You want to be left alone. You do not feel safe in the hospital.

Past medical history

Mild asthma.

Drug history

Salbutamol 100 µg inhaler, 2 puffs PRN.

Social history

- You live with your parents and one brother in a council house but you want to move out because your family are turning against you.
- You do not smoke cigarettes but smoke cannabis around once a week and have done so for several years. You have never been a heavy cannabis user. You do not use any other illicit drugs, or legal highs.
- You drink alcohol occasionally.

Family history

None significant.

Diagnosis

Acute psychotic episode.

Differentials

- Schizophrenia
- Drug-induced psychosis
- Psychosis secondary to a mood disorder
- Schizoaffective disorder
- Organic disorder, e.g. space-occupying lesion
- Delusional disorder.

Station 3

Patient's details

Patient's name: Sandy Williams

Patient's age: 30 years

Patient's occupation: Musician

Presenting complaint

- Your speech is fast and you seem restless and fidgety. You find it difficult to sit still, and spend time pacing during the interview. You also have more eye contact than normal and make flirtatious comments from time to time.
- You do not see anything wrong with playing guitar in your next door neighbour's garden.
- You have been feeling 'over the moon' for the last few weeks and think that everyone else is boring and needs cheering up. You are extremely happy.
- You haven't been having much sleep but still find that you have lots of energy. At most you have had 1–2 hours a night.
- You have been having sex with lots of men recently but have not told your husband. You describe your husband as 'frigid'.
- You have also spent lots of money on things such as clothes and alcohol. You have spent approximately £4000 in the last week.
- You do not have any grandiose delusions.

Ideas, concerns, expectations

You have no insight. You have no concerns as you have never felt better. You want to be left alone.

Past medical history

You suffered from depression 2 months ago.

Drug history

Fluoxetine 20 mg OD over the last 2 months.

Social history

- You live alone after your husband left you 3 days ago for cheating on him. You have no children.
- You do not smoke but drink moderate amounts of alcohol.
- You have never taken any illicit drugs.

Family history

Your mother suffers from bipolar affective disorder.

Diagnosis

Bipolar affective disorder: current episode mania without psychosis.

Differential diagnoses

- Manic episode
- Cyclothymia
- Organic disorder.

Station 4

Patient's details

Patient's name: Amy West

Patient's age: 26 years

Patient's occupation: Bar lady

Presenting complaint

- You took 15 paracetamol tablets in the moments after an argument with your boyfriend. You got extremely scared shortly after you had consumed the tablets and told your boyfriend. You both then immediately went to the hospital.
- The reason you took the tablets was to take your own life to get back at your boyfriend, but you regretted this impulsive act shortly after you consumed the tablets.
- You have never done anything like this before.
- You no longer want to kill yourself but still feel down and depressed about your life. You have no diagnosed psychiatric illness.
- You have never planned to harm or kill yourself and have never written a suicide note.
- You have been feeling quite low in mood for 2 months now and this started ever since your dog, who you were very close to, died. You also feel more tired than before and have not had sex for over a month because your sexual drive has diminished. You feel very lonely because your boyfriend is busy most of the time balancing two jobs, and your family live far away. You haven't told any of your friends because you think that they have their own stress to deal with.
- You are not getting any enjoyment from life, and haven't had an appetite recently.

Ideas, concerns, expectations

You realize that you might be suffering from depression. You are concerned that you will get worse, to a point that you won't want to live any more, but you are willing to accept help. You do not have any current thoughts about ending your life. You want to get well.

Past medical history

None significant.

Drug history

None significant.

Family history

Your mother suffered from depression.

Social history

Live in a flat with your boyfriend and are currently unemployed. You smoke 15 cigarettes a day and drink 21 units of alcohol a week. You do not take illicit drugs.

Diagnosis

Moderate depressive disorder.

Attempted suicide with low risk of follow-up suicide, and no ongoing thoughts to end her life.

Differential diagnosis

- Adjustment disorder
- Acute stress reaction
- Organic cause of depression
- Borderline personality disorder – very unlikely given the information.

Station 5

Patient's details

Patient's name: James Anderson

Patient's age: 50 years

Patient's occupation: Mechanic

Presenting complaint

- You have been persuaded by your wife to come in because you have been drinking more than usual.
- You have been drinking high amounts of alcohol for a number of years. Your drinking began getting out of control 5 years ago. You have drunk daily over the last 3 years, and this has gradually increased. You put this down to stress because of financial difficulties.
- You consume about one 700 ml bottle of vodka (40% alcohol by volume) a day now.
- 6 months ago you were drinking about half this amount.
- You feel shaky and agitated when you don't drink alcohol and drink to prevent this from happening, even if it is first thing in the morning. You often need a drink first thing in the morning in bed, to allow you to get up in the mornings.
- You are aware of the harmful effects of alcohol but still choose to continue drinking. You admit that you have lost control of your drinking, and are drinking more and more to get the same effect.
- You have tried cutting down in the past but have failed to maintain this.
- Your mood has been low but you have no other symptoms of depression.
- Your entire life now revolves around drinking alcohol.
- You have no problems with your memory.

Ideas, concerns, expectations

You are aware that you are an 'alcoholic'.

Past medical history

- Acute pancreatitis (2 years ago).
- You have been told that your 'liver blood tests are abnormal'.

Drug history

Omeprazole 20 mg OD for reflux.

Social history

- You live with your wife and have one child aged 20 who does not live with you.
- You are a self-employed mechanic and your business seems to be having significant financial problems as a result of your drinking.
- You do not smoke and do not take illicit drugs.

Diagnosis

Alcohol dependence syndrome.

Mark schemes

For each station we have developed a checklist, identifying the core aspects of the history and mental state that would need to be covered. At the end of each mark sheet there are a series of questions that the examiner might ask the student. For each competency the examiner will have to identify whether the student has met this in their interaction with the patient, or simulated patient. We have also identified a number of questions that could be asked in a viva situation. Across different universities there will be different mark schemes or competency lists. We have given an indication of what would be expected for a given clinical scenario.

Station 1

Competency level	Yes	Partial	No
Introduction			
Appropriate introduction and checks patient's name			
Explains the purpose of the interview and gains consent			
Presenting complaint and history of presenting complaint			
Starts with an open question and listens without interrupting			
Establishes the onset and course of the low mood			
Enquires about precipitating factors such as stress, life events, current social situation			
Asks about the other core symptoms of depression: anhedonia and lack of energy			
Asks about biological symptoms of depression: difficulty sleeping, weight loss, loss of appetite, loss of libido.			
Asks about cognitive symptoms of depression, e.g. guilt, lack of concentration, hopelessness, negative views of the future and those around them			

Competency level	Yes	Partial	No
Explores possibility of organic symptoms by asking about symptoms of thyroid dysfunction, anaemia, etc.			
Explores possibility of psychotic depression by asking about delusions and hallucinations			
Explores the patient's ideas, concerns and expectations – what does the patient want?			
Risk assessment			
Thoughts about self-harm, suicide, thoughts of harming others			
Past psychiatric history			
Past medical history			
Drug history including allergies			
Relevant family history			
Social history			
Asks about housing circumstances, dependants, occupation			
Asks about alcohol, smoking and substance misuse history			
Communication skills			
Appropriate questioning style (mix of open and closed questions)			
Organized approach to history taking			
Examiner to ask the candidate: What are your differential diagnoses?			
Appropriate differentials: moderate or severe depression, bipolar affective disorder, adjustment disorder, thyroid dysfunction or other organic causes			
Examiner to ask the candidate: What are the causes of depression?			
Candidate provides an organized answer with biological as well as psychosocial causes			
Examiner to ask the candidate: What is an appropriate management plan for the patient?			
Gives an organized answer using the bio-psychosocial model. Antidepressants with SSRI first-line, psychotherapies most notably CBT, social support groups, etc. Lifestyle changes, exercise, healthy diet, consider activity scheduling – voluntary work, adult education, etc.			

Station 2

Competency level	Yes	Partial	No
Introduction			
Appropriate introduction and checks patient's name			
Explains the purpose of the interview and gains consent			
Presenting complaint and history of presenting complaint			
Starts with an open question and listens without interrupting			
Enquires about precipitating factors such as stress, life events that may have led up to this			
Identifies and tests the patient's delusions by asking whether they think their thoughts are unusual			
Screens for other delusional beliefs – persecution, reference, grandiose			
Explores hallucinations in different modalities. Identifies the third person auditory hallucinations in the form of a running commentary			
Asks appropriate follow-up questions regarding the hallucinations, e.g. in what person, how many voices, content of voices			
Asks about thought interference (thought insertion, withdrawal and broadcast)			
Asks about passivity phenomenon			
Enquires about current mood, and a history of depressive and manic episodes. When checking current mood, asks about anhedonia and energy			
Checks the patient's cognition			
Enquires about previous episodes of mental health problems			
Explores the patient's ideas, concerns and expectations			
Risk assessment			
Thoughts about self-harm, suicide, thoughts of harming others			
Past psychiatric history			
Past medical history			
Drug history including allergies			
Relevant family history			
Social history			

Competency level	Yes	Partial	No
Asks about housing circumstances, dependants, occupation			
Asks about alcohol, smoking and substance misuse history			
Communication skills			
Appropriate questioning style (mix of open and closed questions)			
Organized approach to history taking			
Examiner to ask the candidate: What are the differential diagnoses?			
Appropriate differentials: acute psychotic episode, schizophrenia, drug-induced psychosis, psychosis secondary to a mood disorder, delusional disorder, schizoaffective disorder			
Examiner to ask the candidate: What are Schneider's first rank symptoms?			
Thought interference (thought insertion, withdrawal and broadcast), third person auditory hallucinations, delusional perception, and passivity phenomenon			
Examiner to ask the candidate: What are the different types of schizophrenia?			
Paranoid, hebephrenic, post-schizophrenic, catatonic, residual, undifferentiated, simple, mixed			

Station 3

Competency level	Yes	Partial	No
Introduction			
Appropriate introduction and checks patient's name			
Explains the purpose of the interview and gains consent			
Presenting complaint and history of presenting complaint			
Starts with an open question and listens without interrupting			
Enquires about onset, timing and course of the symptoms			
Asks about current mood			
Asks about increased energy and lack of sleep			
Asks about increased libido			
Asks about racing thoughts			
Asks about grandiose delusions			
Asks about passivity phenomenon			

Competency level	Yes	Partial	No
Asks about other types of delusional beliefs			
Asks about hallucinations in a variety of modalities			
Asks appropriate questions to check cognition			
Enquires about previous episodes of mania			
Enquires about previous episodes and treatment for depression			
Explores the patient's ideas, concerns and expectations			
Risk assessment			
Thoughts about self-harm, suicide, thoughts of harming others			
Past psychiatric history			
Past medical history			
Drug history including allergies			
Relevant family history			
Social history			
Asks about housing circumstances, dependants, occupation			
Asks about alcohol, smoking and substance misuse history			
Communication skills			
Appropriate questioning style (mix of open and closed questions)			
Organized approach to history taking			
Examiner to ask the candidate: What are the differential diagnoses?			
Appropriate differentials: bipolar affective disorder current episode mania or hypomania, acute manic episode without psychosis, drug-induced mania, organic disease, cyclothymia			
Examiner to ask the candidate: What is formal thought disorder?			
Candidate recognizes that it refers to abnormalities of the way thoughts are linked together. Candidate gives examples of different types of formal thought disorder, e.g. derailment of thought, tangential thinking, word salad, circumstantiality, thought blocking and neologism			
Examiner to ask the candidate: What is the difference between mania and hypomania?			
Hypomanic episodes must last for several days and do not usually require hospitalization. Hypomania does not involve psychotic features such as grandiose delusions. In mania, symptoms are more severe to the point that the individual's everyday life is significantly impaired and psychotic features may be present			

Station 4

Competency level	Yes	Partial	No
Introduction			
Appropriate introduction and checks patient's name			
Explains the purpose of the interview and gains consent			
Risk assessment			
Starts with an open question and listens without interrupting			
Enquires about onset, timing and course of the mood symptoms			
Asks about precipitating factors for the overdose			
Identifies the steps leading up to the overdose, and then the steps to getting help and coming to hospital			
Asks about current suicidal ideation			
Asks about planning for the suicide attempt			
Asks whether a letter was written beforehand			
Asks about final acts such as writing a will, sorting out finances, etc.			
Asks about attempts to avoid discovery			
Asks about previous suicide attempts			
Asks about self-harm previously			
Explores any current mood disorder symptoms			
Explores history of psychiatric illness, e.g. depression			
Explores other risk factors of suicide			
Explores protective factors			
Explores risk to others			
Explores the patient's ideas, concerns and expectations			
Past medical history			
Drug history including allergies			
Relevant family history			
Social history			
Asks about housing circumstances, dependants, occupation			

Competency level	Yes	Partial	No
Asks about alcohol, smoking and substance misuse history			
Communication skills			
Appropriate questioning style (mix of open and closed questions)			
Organized approach to history taking			
Examiner to ask the candidate: What is the appropriate management plan for this patient?			
Candidate identifies that the patient wishes to seek help. The patient and partner can be seen to discuss going home with support. The patient should be seen by the Crisis Team and have a full psychosocial assessment including a risk assessment. The patient can possibly be home treated. Assessment for depression is needed with a discussion about a bio-psychosocial approach to the management of this.			
Examiner to ask the candidate: What are the risk factors for suicide?			
Candidate gives a number of risk factors (five or more – see Section 9.2, Suicide and risk assessment). An extra mark is given for a structured answer, e.g. divided into clinical and socio-demographic.			
Examiner to ask the candidate: What are the protective factors for suicide, in general, and in this situation?			
Candidate gives a number of protective factors (five or more – see Section 9.2, Suicide and risk assessment).			

Station 5

Competency level	Yes	Partial	No
Introduction			
Appropriate introduction and checks patient's name			
Explains the purpose of the interview and gains consent			
Presenting complaint			
Starts with an open question and listens without interrupting			
Establishes the onset and current level of use of alcohol			
Enquires about precipitating factors such as stress, life events, etc.			
Establishes current amount of alcohol consumed in units			
Explores increased tolerance to alcohol			

Competency level	Yes	Partial	No
Explores withdrawal effects			
Explores compulsive need to drink			
Explores use despite knowledge of harm			
Explores difficulties in control over alcohol			
Explores the importance of alcohol/primacy of alcohol in his life			
Explores narrowed repertoire of drinking			
Asks about mood symptoms			
Asks about delusional beliefs and any visual or auditory hallucinations			
Explores any cognitive symptoms			
Explores the patient's ideas, concerns and expectations			
Risk assessment			
Thoughts about self-harm, suicide, thoughts of harming others			
Past medical history			
Drug history including allergies			
Relevant family history			
Social history			
Asks about housing circumstances, dependants, occupation			
Asks about smoking and substance misuse history			
Communication skills			
Appropriate questioning style (mix of open and closed questions)			
Organized approach to history taking			
Examiner to ask the student: Does the patient have alcohol dependence syndrome, and if so, why?			
Candidate identifies that the patient has alcohol dependence syndrome and gives evidence to back this up			

Competency level	Yes	Partial	No
Examiner to ask the student: What drug is used for alcohol detoxification and how is this prescribed? What other medication could be appropriate?			
Candidate identifies that a benzodiazepine is used, e.g. chlordiazepoxide and this is given as a tapering dose orally, over approximately 7 days. Candidate also identifies the importance of vitamin B replacement, orally with thiamine, or possibly with IV vitamin B replacement. Identifies the importance of this to prevent Wernicke's encephalopathy/Korsakoff's psychosis			
Examiner to ask the candidate: What are the long-term solutions to alcohol misuse for this patient?			
Candidate gives an organized answer giving both pharmacological (disulfiram, acamprosate, naltrexone) and psychosocial (motivational interviewing and support groups such as Alcoholics Anonymous) management options			

Chapter 15

Exam-style questions

1. A 24-year-old patient presents to the Emergency Department. During the mental state examination he describes hearing the voices of three individuals outside his flat. He has never been able to see these individuals. The three individuals talk about him, and the patient has heard them plotting to kill him. On several occasions he heard a presenter on Radio 1 talk to him, mention his name, and threaten to kill him.

    What symptoms are described in the scenario?
    A. Auditory pseudo-hallucinations and delusions of reference.
    B. Second and third person auditory hallucinations.
    C. Second person auditory hallucinations and delusions of reference.
    D. Third person auditory hallucinations and delusions of reference.
    E. Third person auditory hallucinations and persecutory delusions.

2. A 56-year-old woman presents to her general practitioner with a 3-week history of low mood. She is waking up at 4am, and is unable to get back to sleep. She normally gets out of bed at 7am, she has lost her appetite and is not interested in food. She denies any suicidal thoughts and does not feel hopeless for the future. She used to enjoy walking her dog and going to the gym, but hasn't felt like doing this. Six weeks ago her mother who she was very close to passed away after a long illness.

    What is the most appropriate diagnosis?
    A. Adjustment disorder.
    B. Bereavement reaction.
    C. Mild depressive episode.
    D. Moderate depressive episode.
    E. Severe depressive episode.

3. A 22-year-old man presents to the Emergency Department. He has been taken there by friends from university who are concerned about his behaviour. He has not been sleeping for the last 7 days. He is talking extremely quickly and it is difficult to follow his conversation. He tells the junior doctor that his blood has healing powers, and offers to use this to help staff in the department. He appears elated in mood.

    What is the most appropriate diagnosis?
    A. Bipolar affective disorder, current episode mania with psychosis.
    B. Bipolar affective disorder, current episode mania without psychosis.
    C. Hypomanic episode.
    D. Mania with psychosis.
    E. Mania without psychosis.

4. A 16-year-old male is taken to his GP by his mother. He has been socially withdrawn for 2 weeks and has been very frightened. He confides in the GP that for the last 2 weeks he has been concerned that his neighbours are talking about him. He can hear them outside his bedroom. He is worried that they can see everything that he does, as they talk about everything he does in the house.

He believes that there must be cameras in the house, and he has been looking for these over the last 2 weeks. He has suffered with depression in the past, but his mood is currently euthymic. He has smoked cannabis in the past. The last occasion was 3 weeks ago with some friends.

What is the most appropriate diagnosis?

A. Acute schizophrenia-like psychotic disorder.
B. Delusional disorder.
C. Paranoid schizophrenia.
D. Schizoaffective disorder.
E. Severe depressive episode with psychosis.

5. **A 50-year-old with known paranoid schizophrenia reported that on the way to see his sister he suddenly had a desire to go to a fast food restaurant. He had never eaten there before. He believes that the thought about going to a fast food restaurant is not his own. He becomes worried that it may be a trap where some harm will come to him if he goes to the fast food restaurant.**

What is the symptom described above?

A. Delusion of reference.
B. Persecutory delusion.
C. Thought broadcast.
D. Thought insertion.
E. Thought withdrawal.

6. **A 26-year-old woman presents to her GP. She is extremely worried about a presentation she is due to give at work in the coming weeks. She has never felt comfortable giving presentations. She also states that she does not like going out and eating in public, and worries that she may vomit. She describes herself as quiet and shy and lacking in confidence around others. When she gets worried she complains that she blushes excessively, starts to feel hot and sweaty, and shakes. This can last for 10 to 30 minutes depending on the situation. In the past she has always found a reason not to give presentations.**

What is the most likely diagnosis?

A. Generalized anxiety disorder.
B. Panic disorder with agoraphobia.
C. Panic disorder without agoraphobia.
D. Social phobia.
E. Vomiting phobia.

7. **A 47-year-old man presents to the GP complaining of recurrent episodes of chest pain. These episodes can happen at any time of the day or night, and the pain is not made worse on exertion. He explains that when the chest pain starts he becomes convinced that he will die. He has called an ambulance and been to the Emergency Department on five occasions over the last month. When the chest pain starts he complains of breathlessness, chest tightness, tingling in his fingers, and a feeling of being lightheaded. He has worried that he will pass out. These**

episodes can last for up to an hour. When seen in the Emergency Department he has had blood tests and an ECG, and there has been no evidence of a cardiac cause for his problems. Between episodes he feels well, and has no other physical or mental health concerns. The last three episodes all occurred when he was out shopping, and he has avoided going back to the supermarket, in case it happens again. He has continued to go to work.

What would be the appropriate treatment in primary care?

A.   Cognitive behavioural therapy.

B.   Further investigations including ECG.

C.   Refer on for psychiatric review within a community mental health team.

D.   Short course of benzodiazepines, and advice to stop avoiding situations causing anxiety.

E.   Watch and wait and see again in 2–4 weeks in primary care.

8.   An 18-year-old man is brought to see his GP by his parents. They are concerned about his behaviour. It takes him 2 hours to get ready in the morning. He has a very set routine, including cleaning the bathroom, and then washing himself. He explains he has to clean himself in a particular way, and finishes by washing his hands 11 times. The cleaning routine takes him about 2 hours. If he is interrupted he has to start the routine from the very beginning. The skin on his hands is very dry and scaly. He gets very frustrated by his cleaning, and wishes he didn't have to do this. He accepts that he is not dirty or contaminated. If he tries to resist he becomes distressed and describes multiple unpleasant physical symptoms of anxiety. He continues to worry that he is dirty, and washes his hands throughout the day. When he gets home, he has to take off his clothes immediately and put these in the washing machine before showering again. He has tried to make his parents do the same thing in case they are contaminated, but they have so far refused. The GP thinks he has an obsessive–compulsive disorder.

Which of the following is most important when making this diagnosis?

A.   Asking about a family history of obsessive–compulsive disorder.

B.   Checking that the patient believes the thoughts are his own.

C.   Checking the core and other symptoms of depression.

D.   Checking the patient's insight into his presentation.

E.   The symptoms need to have been present for 1 week.

9.   A 21-year-old complains that since a car accident where he was driving, he has not been able to get back in a car, either as a driver or as a passenger. No one was seriously hurt in the accident, although his car was written off. When he goes to get in a car he complains of multiple symptoms of anxiety. The accident happened 3 months ago, and the problems are not getting any easier. The man has read about post-traumatic stress disorder and wonders if he has this.

What features (other than those described above) would you need to check to clarify this diagnosis?

A.   Flashbacks to the accident, insomnia, startle reaction.

B.   Flashbacks to the accident, low mood and nightmares.

C.   Flashbacks to the accident, nightmares, insomnia, and anhedonia.

D. Flashbacks to the accident, startle reaction and nightmares.

E. Flashbacks to the accident, startle reaction, low mood, insomnia.

10. **A 35-year-old woman presents to her GP with a 3-month history of gradually worsening low mood, anhedonia and being easily fatigued. She has been off work for 1 week, as she has struggled to get out of bed. She appears unkempt and is quietly spoken. Her speech is not very spontaneous, but she does answer questions when asked. She feels that she is a bad person and is being punished for letting her partner down. Her partner has brought her to the doctor for help. She is struggling to eat and has lost 10 kg in weight. She does manage to sleep, but wakes up repeatedly during the night. She needs to be encouraged to shower. She denies any active suicidal thoughts but states she deserves to be dead. She cannot concentrate for very long, and during the brief consultation, a lot of the history has to come from the partner. She has no history of mental or physical health problems.**

What is the most appropriate treatment?

A. Offer an antipsychotic for her beliefs about needing to be punished.

B. Offer sertraline (an SSRI).

C. Offer lofepramine (a TCA).

D. Refer for urgent CBT treatment in primary care.

E. Watch and wait and see in clinic in 2 weeks' time.

11. **A 33-year-old man is being seen by a psychiatrist in clinic. He has had three previous admissions with mania. On two of these occasions he was found by the police naked in public, trying to gain access to Parliament. On these two occasions he stated that he was the Prime Minister of England, and needed to make a speech. The last admission for mania was approximately 1 year ago. He understands that he has bipolar affective disorder. He presents in clinic today with a 3-week history of low mood. He has never had an episode of depression before. He rates his mood as 0 out of 10, and is extremely tearful. He has multiple symptoms of depression and is diagnosed with severe depression. He is referred to the home treatment team as he has some suicidal thoughts. He is currently taking olanzapine 10 mg (an oral antipsychotic) which has treated his mania.**

What would be the most appropriate treatment?

A. Duloxetine (SNRI).

B. Lamotrigine (anti-epileptic and mood stabilizer).

C. Lofepramine (TCA).

D. Sertraline (SSRI).

E. Sertraline (SSRI) and cognitive behavioural therapy (CBT).

12. **A 33-year-old man presents to the Emergency Department. He is brought there by his wife. He has a 4-week history of a severe depressive disorder. He has been depressed once before 3 years ago, and during that episode he tried to hang himself. Over the last 6 months his antidepressants have been reduced and stopped. He is again presenting with low mood, rating his mood as 0 out of 10. He feels hopeless about the future. On questioning he states that he wishes he**

were dead and has bought a rope and has planned to hang himself. He cannot see any other way out of his current situation. He also states that he has bankrupted his family, and he deserves to die. His wife states that this is not the case. During his last episode of depression he was treated for a depression with psychosis with antidepressants and antipsychotics. He passively accepts whatever treatment is offered as he believes he will die whatever is done, and that no one can help him. His wife is extremely distressed. She is also the main carer for their 3 children aged, 6 years, 3 years and 6 months.

As the Emergency Department junior doctor you make a referral to the out of hours psychiatry team. What do you feel would be an appropriate treatment?

A. Admission following a Mental Health Act assessment for assessment and treatment.
B. Admission informally to a psychiatry ward for assessment and treatment.
C. Discharge home, with a letter to the GP to refer on for psychiatry support, and advice about starting antidepressants.
D. Discharge home with a prescription for antidepressants and antipsychotics and a follow up appointment in psychiatry outpatients.
E. Discharge home with a referral to the local community mental health team for outpatient follow-up and support.

13. **A 16-year-old is brought to the GP by her parents. She is extremely thin, and has been dieting for the last 4 years. She has yet to enter puberty. She is 1.6 m tall and weighs 42 kg. She continues to worry that she is fat and is trying to lose more weight. She limits her food intake to 400 calories a day, and exercises for 2 hours each day.**
    What is her BMI?
    A. 10.3
    B. 13.125
    C. 14.5
    D. 16.4
    E. 26.3

14. **A 23-year-old woman presents to the Emergency Department having vomited fresh red blood. During the history she reports that she has been making herself vomit on a regular basis for the last 5 years. She is worried about putting on weight and is concerned that she is fat. Her height is 1.6 m, and she weighs 53 kg. She describes periods of time where she eats large quantities of food, followed by episodes of induced vomiting. She also abuses laxatives on a daily basis and exercises excessively. She is clear that she needs to lose at least 5 kg before she will be happy with her weight. She has very low self-esteem, and eats for comfort.**
    What is the most likely diagnosis?
    A. Anorexia nervosa.
    B. Atypical anorexia nervosa.
    C. Bulimia nervosa.
    D. Eating disorder not otherwise specified (EDNOS).
    E. Overeating associated with other psychological disturbances.

15. **A 29-year-old woman suddenly comes to at Peterborough station while buying a coffee. She is fully dressed. She lives in Leicester, and does not recall waking that morning, nor how she travelled to Peterborough. She has no reason to visit Peterborough. This has never happened before.**
    What is the most likely diagnosis?
    A. Dissociative amnesia.
    B. Dissociative fugue.
    C. Dissociative stupor.
    D. Factitious disorder.
    E. Malingering.

16. **A 49-year-old man presents repeatedly to see his GP. He is complaining of abdominal pain, which is intermittent. This is central in nature and is referred through to his back. Occasionally the pain is associated with a feeling of being bloated and intermittent diarrhoea. There is no blood or mucus when he goes to the toilet. He has had a number of investigations for this, but to date, there are no positive clinical findings.**
    If we presume that there is no physical cause for this presentation what is the most likely diagnosis?
    A. Delusional disorder (hypochondriacal).
    B. Factitious disorder.
    C. Hypochondriacal disorder.
    D. Malingering.
    E. Somatization disorder.

17. **A 36-year-old man is brought to the Emergency Department. He has been in the department four times before in the last 6 months, and it is known that he has alcohol dependence. There is a concern that he has developed Wernicke's encephalopathy.**
    What are the signs and symptoms of this disorder?
    A. Ataxia, clouding of consciousness, disorientation to time, peripheral neuropathy.
    B. Ophthalmoplegia, nystagmus, ataxia, clouding of consciousness.
    C. Ophthalmoplegia, nystagmus, clouding of consciousness, short-term memory loss.
    D. Ophthalmoplegia, nystagmus, ataxia, disorientation to time.
    E. Nystagmus, ataxia, short-term memory loss, peripheral neuropathy.

18. **A 47-year-old patient is admitted to a medical assessment unit with haematemesis. He is known to drink 6 litres of strong white cider each day and has been drinking this heavily for about 12 months. Within 4 hours of admission he begins to sweat and shake.**
    What treatment is appropriate for his alcohol problems?
    A. Gradually reducing doses of benzodiazepines over 5–7 days with oral thiamine and vitamin B.
    B. Gradually reducing doses of benzodiazepines over 5–7 days with Pabrinex injections.
    C. Low dose benzodiazepines for 1–2 days with oral thiamine and vitamin B.

D. Low dose benzodiazepines for 1–2 days with Pabrinex injections.

E. Low dose benzodiazepines for 5–7 days with Pabrinex injections.

19. **A 21-year-old intravenous heroin user is admitted with a groin abscess. He has been injecting and smoking heroin since the age of 15 on a daily basis. He rapidly starts to demonstrate symptoms of heroin withdrawal.**

Apart from withdrawal, what other features make up the dependence syndrome?

A. Compulsion to take the substance, evidence of tolerance, spending significant amounts on the substance, continuing to take the substance despite evidence of harm.

B. Compulsion to take the substance, evidence of tolerance, neglect of alternative pleasures, continuing to take the substance despite evidence of harm, inability to control substance use.

C. Compulsion to take the substance, evidence of tolerance, neglect of alternative pleasures, continuing to take the substance despite evidence of harm, spending significant amounts on the substance.

D. Compulsion to take the substance, evidence of tolerance, neglect of alternative pleasures, spending significant amounts on the substance.

E. Compulsion to take the substance, evidence of tolerance, spending significant amounts on the substance, inability to control substance misuse.

20. **A 50-year-old man is found collapsed in a public place. During the admission it is clear that he has no friends or family, and has been living alone since his early twenties. He has lost contact with his family, and has no wish for social contact. He has worked for nearly 30 years in a warehouse. He appears cold and detached, and does not report that he has any particular interests. He watches television, and occasionally goes cycling. He is dressed appropriately but takes little interest in his appearance. There is no history of any psychotic or affective symptoms. His collapse was caused by an undiagnosed medical condition. He has not seen his GP in the last 10 years.**

What could the diagnosis be in this situation?

A. Autism spectrum disorder.

B. Paranoid personality disorder.

C. Paranoid schizophrenia.

D. Schizoid personality disorder.

E. Social phobia.

21. **A 20-year-old man is seen in the Emergency Department. He has a fracture to his 5th metacarpal on the left hand. He has been in an altercation with two other youths. He is impatient to be seen and staff report that he has been intimidating. When he is told he has to wait he loses his temper and the security guards are called. He has been seen in the department before, and on reading this report it is clear he has a significant forensic history. He has been convicted of affray and actual bodily harm on numerous occasions. He has a history of poly-substance misuse and drinks alcohol heavily on a social basis. He was permanently excluded from several schools because of his behaviour, including assaults on teachers and staff. He has a history of self-harm through cutting, dating back to early teens.**

When seen he reports he got into a fight at a bar because he didn't like how the two youths looked. He blamed them for the fight, as he states they shouldn't have been in the bar. He wants to leave to see his girlfriend. They have been together 3 months, and she is 6 weeks pregnant. She had been with him at the bar, and had threatened to leave him when the fight started. The police arrive in the department to see him about the fight. He is rude and dismissive about the police, and doesn't appear to be worried about the situation.

In ICD-10 terms what is the most likely diagnosis?

A. Antisocial personality disorder.
B. Borderline personality disorder.
C. Dissocial personality disorder.
D. Emotionally unstable personality disorder.
E. Paranoid personality disorder.

22. A 23-year-old woman presents to the Emergency Department with a self-inflicted cut to her left arm. She is well known to the department with a 6-year history of regular self-harm through cutting. She tells staff she has had an argument with her mother and was distressed. She uses self-harm to help her manage and relieve tension and distress. She has presented to the Emergency Department on approximately 30 occasions in the last 12 months. She states that the cut was not an attempt to end her life. She requires 15 stitches, and asks to be discharged from hospital. She has no immediate thoughts to self-harm, but states that if the argument continues she may self-harm again to relieve tension. She is seen by the on-call psychiatrist in the Emergency Department. She is having weekly group psychotherapy and sees a consultant psychiatrist in the outpatient clinic every 6 weeks, and is due to be seen in 5 days' time.

What would be an appropriate course of action?

A. Consider admission to a psychiatric hospital.
B. Discharge home and counsel about immediately stopping self-harm.
C. Discharge home and refer for community mental health team input.
D. Discharge home with a letter to the psychiatrist and psychotherapist.
E. Discharge home with a prescription of benzodiazepines as an alternative way of managing distress/tension.

23. A 70-year-old man is admitted to the medical assessment unit. He has a 5-day history of coughing up green sputum, and being increasingly short of breath with oxygen saturations on air of 86%. He is not known to have COPD. His only other significant past medical history is a 1-year history of Alzheimer's disease. He has been living with his wife, and before admission was independent with his activities of daily living. During the first night in a bay with five patients he becomes agitated and appears extremely confused. He tells the doctor and staff to get out of his house. He is disoriented in time. He appears to be visually hallucinating.

What would be the most appropriate treatment?

A. Ensure he remains on oxygen and prescribe 10 mg haloperidol for his agitation and ask nursing staff to stay with him to provide reassurance.

B. Ensure he remains on oxygen, move him to a well-lit side room, and prescribe 10 mg haloperidol for his agitation.
C. Ensure he remains on oxygen, move him to a well-lit side room, ask nursing staff to talk slowly and calmly to him to provide reassurance.
D. Ensure he remains on oxygen, move him to a side room to avoid distress to other patients, and prescribe benzodiazepines for his agitation.
E. Ensure he remains on oxygen, prescribe benzodiazepines for his agitation and ask nursing staff to stay with him to provide reassurance.

24. **An 85-year-old woman presents to her GP. She reports that she is losing items in her house and is concerned about her short-term memory. She complains that she is becoming increasingly forgetful. On formal testing she struggles with orientation to time and short-term memory. She scores 23 out of 30 on the Mini-Mental State Examination. Family report that her memory has deteriorated over the last 12 months. She has never smoked. She has a history of hypertension, but no other significant medical or family history. Her physical examination is unremarkable. She recalls an incident one night several weeks ago when she thought she heard something in her garden. It was 4am, and she got up and looked out of her bedroom window. She thinks she might have seen someone lurking in a bush, but she is not sure. She recalls going downstairs and turning the outside light on, but no-one was there. She admits to drinking one bottle of white wine (11%, 750 ml) each week.**
If she does have an early dementia what is the most likely diagnosis?
A. Alcoholic dementia.
B. Alzheimer's disease.
C. Frontal lobe dementia.
D. Lewy body dementia.
E. Vascular dementia.

25. **A 60-year-old patient presents with a 30-year history of heavy alcohol dependence. He is currently drinking on a daily basis. He is drinking 5 L of strong white cider each day (10% ABV) and a 700 ml bottle of vodka (40% ABV) each day.**
How many units of alcohol does he drink each day?
A. 22.5
B. 28
C. 43
D. 50
E. 78

26. **A 21-year-old woman is being cared for in a learning disability home. She has had difficulties since birth, including some motor problems. She is able to express her basic needs, and needs support with all aspects of personal care. Her IQ is tested and found to be 45. She has poorly controlled epilepsy with regular tonic–clonic seizures.**
How would you classify her intellectual disability?
A. Mild intellectual disability.

B. Moderate intellectual disability.
C. Pervasive developmental disorder.
D. Profound intellectual disability.
E. Severe intellectual disability.

27. **A 17-year-old man is brought to the GP by his mother. While his mother has no major concerns, there have been ongoing problems with his behaviour reported by his school. He has always struggled to make friends easily, and has been in a few fights at school when other students have objected to comments he has made. He struggles to understand other people's motivations, and has a limited range of interests. He cannot show or feign interests in other hobbies, or people. He is interested in a particular comic which he has collected for the last 5 years. He always carries some of these with him, and unless distracted will start reading these. He has done well at GCSEs in some subjects that he is interested in, getting 1 A*, 2 As, 2 Bs, 3 Cs and 2 Ds. The school find that he is very inflexible, and struggles with any change. He has no close friends.**
What could be your preferred diagnosis to explore?
A. Asperger's syndrome.
B. Depressive disorder.
C. Dissocial personality disorder.
D. Prodromal phase of a psychotic disorder.
E. Schizoid personality disorder.

28. **An 18-year-old man presents with a first episode of psychosis. He has third person auditory hallucinations in the form of a running commentary, and has persecutory delusions. He has been threatening towards people he believes are trying to kill him and he is admitted to hospital. There is no history of substance misuse. He is started on oral risperidone.**
What investigations would be appropriate before starting antipsychotics?
A. ECG and blood glucose.
B. ECG and blood glucose and lipids.
C. Full blood count and an ECG.
D. Full blood count, blood glucose and lipids.
E. Full blood count, urea and electrolytes and liver function tests.

29. **A 27-year-old woman with a treatment-resistant depression is advised and agreed to start on lithium carbonate. She is also prescribed venlafaxine and mirtazapine. After 3 months her mood improves on this combination.**
What regular blood tests are needed while on this new medication?
A. Full blood count, thyroid function tests and lithium levels.
B. Full blood count, urea and electrolytes and liver function tests.
C. Liver function tests, thyroid function tests and lithium levels.
D. Urea and electrolytes, liver function tests, thyroid function tests and lithium levels.
E. Urea and electrolytes, thyroid function tests and lithium levels.

30. **A 49-year-old man is being prepared for ECT for treatment-resistant depression. He is not eating and drinking without prompting as a result of severe depression. He has not responded to oral antidepressants. He has agreed to have ECT, as this has been effective for him in a previous episode of severe depression. He has a number of physical investigations to prepare him for the general anaesthetic.**
    What would be an absolute contraindication for proceeding with this treatment?
    A. A recent myocardial infarction.
    B. Cardiac arrhythmia.
    C. Cerebral aneurysm.
    D. High anaesthetic risk.
    E. Raised intracranial pressure.

31. **A 23-year-old man is in hospital for the third time. The three admissions have had a similar picture. He becomes convinced that his neighbours have installed cameras in his flat and are watching everything he is doing. He hears the neighbours talking about him and commenting on his actions. On each occasion he has been threatening towards the neighbours. On the first admission he did not respond to oral olanzapine, but did get somewhat better on quetiapine and was discharged home. He was re-admitted 4 weeks later. During the second admission it was clear that he was not improving on quetiapine and he was changed to an atypical depot antipsychotic, and some of his symptoms improved, although he remained paranoid. He was discharged on the depot which he accepted, but he became increasingly unwell despite maximum doses of the depot injection. This was changed to a different atypical depot antipsychotic which he was on for 4 months before the third admission. He has repeatedly been offered cognitive behavioural therapy for psychosis but does not want to proceed with this.**
    What is the next appropriate step in treatment?
    A. Trial of cognitive behavioural therapy while in hospital.
    B. Trial of a depot typical antipsychotic such as Depixol.
    C. Trial of a different atypical antipsychotic such as amisulpride.
    D. Trial of an oral typical antipsychotic such as haloperidol.
    E. Trial of oral clozapine.

32. **A 31-year-old woman presents to her GP. She has a long history of a poorly controlled generalized anxiety disorder with a recurrent depressive disorder. She is currently prescribed sertraline (an SSRI) for depression and anxiety, sodium valproate (as a mood stabilizer), pregabalin (an anti-epileptic used in her situation for anxiety), lorazepam (an anxiolytic), and propranolol (a beta-blocker sometimes used in anxiety). She describes an overwhelming desire to take one of these drugs, and admits to buying it over the internet, as well as taking those prescribed by her GP. When she doesn't take this substance she sweats, shakes and feels physically unwell. She has noticed that in the year that she has been taking this drug she has needed larger doses to make her feel better, and treat her anxiety symptoms.**

Which of the following drugs is she describing and is causing these problems?

A. Lorazepam.
B. Pregabalin.
C. Propranolol.
D. Sertraline.
E. Sodium valproate.

33. A patient presents to the Emergency Department in Birmingham. They have been brought by their parents concerned about their mental health. You are the junior doctor in the department. There is one consultant and a full team of emergency department nursing staff and health care assistants. There are also three security guards in the department. The patient is a 22-year-old man who has taken a significant overdose. He reports that there are people outside the department who have been following him for 3 days. He can hear them now talking about him. They have made threats to kill him and they told him to take the overdose to end his life. There is no evidence of an affective disorder (depression or bipolar). He still believes he needs to 'sacrifice himself.' He accepts physical treatment for his overdose but repeatedly states he wants to leave the Emergency Department to end his life. The on-call psychiatrist is assessing a patient in a police station 20 miles away and will not be with you for 1 hour.
What actions can you and the team in the Emergency Department take?

A. Ask the nurses to detain him using Section 5(4) of the Mental Health Act, which allows his detention for up to 6 hours.
B. If you assess his capacity, and deem him to lack capacity, in his best interests you could ask security to prevent him from leaving until the psychiatrist arrives.
C. Legally you have to allow him to leave the department and ask his parents to keep him under close observation.
D. The Emergency Department consultant can detain him using Section 5(2) of the Mental Health Act which allows his detention for up to 72 hours.
E. You as the junior doctor can detain him using Section 5(2) of the Mental Health Act which allows his detention for up to 72 hours.

34. A 30-year-old woman is in labour. She has a significant needle phobia. During the delivery there are complications, and she requires a Caesarean section to save her life and the life of her baby. She initially consents to the operation. In theatre she subsequently refuses to have the procedure. She has a panic attack when anyone approaches her with a needle, and states she cannot have the procedure. She is extremely distressed by the situation and has multiple symptoms of anxiety. Her husband tells the treating team to perform the Caesarean section. A mental capacity assessment is performed.
What do you think should happen?

A. She is deemed to have capacity and no action is taken.
B. She is deemed to have capacity but the procedure must legally happen to save her baby.

C. She is deemed to lack capacity and in her best interests and in the best interests of the baby the operation should proceed to save her.
D. She is deemed to lack capacity and in her best interests the operation should proceed to save her.
E. She is deemed to lack capacity and therefore her husband can make decisions for her as next of kin, and therefore the operation should proceed.

35. A 69-year-old woman is admitted to the Emergency Department. She is struggling to communicate. She is extremely low in mood, and has been getting worse over the last 6 months since her husband died. She has no physical health problems. She has no enjoyment from life and describes feeling exhausted. She states her husband died suddenly in a car accident. She states that she is responsible for the car accident, although she was not there at the time. She took a large overdose of various medications earlier today with the intention to end her life. Her daughter visited today, found her and alerted the ambulance services. Her daughter reports that her mother has lost a lot of weight, has not been looking after herself or the house, and has been struggling to sleep. The patient wishes to leave hospital and be allowed to die at home. The medication taken includes a lethal dose of paracetamol. The patient does not want the overdose treated medically. She feels that she has no future without her husband. She previously enjoyed spending time with her grandchildren, gardening, socializing with friends, and holidays, none of which she has done for 4 months. Her daughter insists that her mother is treated and is the legal next of kin.
You perform a capacity assessment. What are your options?
A. Admit her to a medical ward and try to persuade her to have treatment. If you cannot persuade her to have treatment for the overdose offer palliative care on the ward.
B. Allow her to leave hospital and die at home as these are her wishes.
C. As the daughter is next of kin you can act on her wishes in this difficult situation.
D. In her best interests treat the overdose and organize aftercare.
E. Organize a Mental Health Act assessment and treat the overdose when detained under the Mental Health Act.

36. A 75-year-old woman has been in a residential home specializing in dementia for the past 3 years. She has a known diagnosis of Alzheimer's disease and her current Mini-Mental State Examination is 8 out of 30. Her husband died 3 years ago prompting the admission to the home, but she is visited by her children and grandchildren. Until recently there have been no management issues in the home. Over the last 3 months she has not engaged in any activities that she used to. She has been less talkative, and has been lashing out at staff when they try to support her with her activities of daily living. She has been wandering in the home and has been tearful on occasions. She has been increasingly difficult for staff to manage. There has not been a marked deterioration in her memory. She is struggling to sleep and from the early hours of the morning is wandering the home, and is aggressive to staff when they try to get her back into bed. Her GP has seen her

and examined her physically. There are no new clinical findings. All of her routine bloods and urinalysis are normal. She is known to have hypertension and type 2 diabetes, but both of these are well controlled. She is a lifelong non-smoker and drinks alcohol very occasionally. Her family are continuing to visit but are clearly distressed. Her daughter is also concerned that in the last 3 months her mother has not been eating well and has lost a substantial amount of weight. She is currently only prescribed donepezil for Alzheimer's, and is on no other psychiatric medication. She has been on this for 4 years.

She is seen by an old age psychiatrist. What might be an appropriate pharmacological treatment?

A. A low dose of an oral antipsychotic to calm her when agitated and distressed, but not on a regular basis.

B. An oral benzodiazepine to treat her agitation.

C. A selective serotonin reuptake inhibitor.

D. Changing her anti-Alzheimer's medication to a different one.

E. Night-time sedation such as zopiclone to help her to sleep.

37. A 45-year-old patient is seen in a psychiatric clinic. He talks about the 'omnimicrotask' but is unable to describe this in detail. He is known to have paranoid schizophrenia. When asked a question he repeats the last syllable of the last word in the sentence repeatedly.

What two symptoms are described above?

A. Neologisms, circumstantiality.

B. Neologisms, knight's move thinking.

C. Neologisms, perseveration.

D. Perseveration, circumstantiality.

E. Perseveration, dysarthria.

38. A 14-year-old boy with a mild learning disability is seen by his new GP. He is attending a special school. He has an autism spectrum disorder, an elongated face, large protruding ears, macro-orchidism, and social anxiety. The GP does not have access to the previous medical records.

What syndrome is most likely?

A. Asperger's syndrome.

B. Down's syndrome.

C. Fragile X syndrome.

D. Klinefelter's syndrome.

E. Prader–Willi syndrome.

39. A 27-year-old woman with schizophrenia is prescribed a typical antipsychotic depot, due to repeated admissions with non-compliance to oral medication. She has now been on this medication for 9 months. She responds well to the treatment and her psychotic symptoms are well controlled. She presents to see her psychiatrist. She reports that she has not had a menstrual cycle for 6 months, whereas before she had regular periods. She also reports that she is getting a

milky discharge from her breasts. The psychiatrist suspects the depot is causing these symptoms and requests a blood test to confirm.

Which dopaminergic pathway is implicated in the side effects above?

A. Basal forebrain cholinergic.
B. Mesocortical.
C. Mesolimbic.
D. Nigrostriatal.
E. Tuberoinfundibular.

40. An 83-year-old single man is seen in the memory clinic by a consultant psychiatrist. He has been struggling at home for 6 months and has had a deteriorating memory. He is accompanied by his son to the clinic. He has no other medical conditions relevant to the memory problems but does have rheumatoid arthritis. The CT brain scan demonstrates marked hippocampal atrophy and his MMSE is 20 out of 30 on the last two clinic visits. He is fiercely independent and does not want to consider any day groups. He has accepted a small package of care. He is struggling to wash and dress in the morning, and is having difficulty making hot drinks. An OT from the community mental health team sees him at home and believes some of his problems relate to his rheumatoid arthritis. He cannot get in and out of the bath, but does not want the bath turned into a shower. He sees his GP on a regular basis for the monitoring of his arthritis. He has appointments with the rheumatologist several times a year, and has had intermittent input from the physiotherapists both in the community and in outpatient settings.

Which professional would be best placed to coordinate his care?

A. General practitioner.
B. Occupational therapist.
C. Physiotherapist.
D. Psychiatrist.
E. Rheumatologist.

Glossary of terms

Acute intoxication: Physiological and psychological response due to the administration of a psychoactive substance.

Affect: Refers to the transient flow of emotion in response to a particular stimulus, i.e. the immediate expression of emotions.

Agnosia: Impaired recognition of sensory stimuli not attributed to sensory loss or language disturbance. May be a feature of dementia.

Akathisia: Unpleasant feeling of restlessness. May be a side effect of antipsychotics.

Amenorrhoea: The absence of menstruation. May be a feature of anorexia nervosa.

Amnesia: A deficit in memory. A feature of organic disorders such as dementia and delirium. Anterograde amnesia is diminished ability to form new memories and retrograde amnesia involves loss of memories of events that have occurred in the past.

Anergia: A lack of energy (core feature of depression).

Anhedonia: A lack of interest in things which were previously enjoyable to the patient.

Anticipatory anxiety: Anxiety at the prospect of encountering the feared situation.

Anxiety: An unpleasant emotional state involving subjective fear and somatic symptoms.

Apathy: Lack of interest, enthusiasm or concern.

Apraxia: Inability to carry out previously learned purposeful movements despite normal coordination and strength. May be a feature of dementia.

Autonomic arousal: A general state of physiological arousal associated with what is commonly referred to as the 'fight or flight syndrome'. Mediated by the sympathetic nervous system with features including sweating, dry mouth and tachycardia.

Beck's triad: A feature of depressive disorder with negative feelings about the self, the world and the future.

Bereavement: Reaction in response to loss of a loved one which may be normal or abnormal.

Bingeing: A feature of bulimia nervosa where patients overeat.

Blunted affect: Reduced expression of emotion.

Body mass index (BMI): A measure of weight relative to height. Calculated as weight (kg) ÷ [height (m)]^2.

Briquet's syndrome: Multiple, recurrent and frequently changing physical symptoms not explained by a physical illness (also known as somatization disorder).

Capgras' syndrome: Delusion that a familiar person has been replaced by an exact duplicate.

Catatonia: Abnormality of tone, posture or movement arising from a disturbed mental state, typically schizophrenia. Can be excessive or decreased motor activity.

Circumstantiality: Thinking progresses slowly as a result of many unnecessary digressions but it eventually returns to original point.

Clang association: Ideas related only by similar or rhyming sounds rather than meaning.

Cognition: Consists of consciousness, orientation, attention, concentration and memory.

Cognitive behavioural therapy: A psychotherapy used to help individuals identify and challenge their negative thoughts and then to modify any abnormal underlying core beliefs.

Compulsions: Repetitive, purposeful behaviours or mental acts that a person feels driven into performing.

Confabulation: Gaps in memory which are unconsciously filled with false memories.

Conversion: Distressing events are transformed into physical symptoms. A feature of dissociative disorder.

Cotard's syndrome (nihilism): Delusion that everything is non-existent including themselves.

Counter-transference: In psychodynamic therapy, refers to the therapist's emotions and attitudes towards the patient.

Da Costa's syndrome: Symptoms of autonomic arousal are attributed by the patient to a disorder of the cardiovascular system (a type of somatoform autonomic dysfunction).

De Clérambault's syndrome: Delusion that an exalted or famous person is in love with them.

Déjà vu: The illusion that an event or experience has already been experienced in the past.

Deliberate self-harm: Refers to an intentional act of self-poisoning or self-injury.

Delirium: An acute, transient, global organic disorder of central nervous system functioning resulting in impaired consciousness and attention.

Delirium tremens: A withdrawal delirium after alcohol cessation, characterized by cognitive impairment, delusions, hallucinations and autonomic arousal.

Delusion: A fixed false belief, which is firmly held, despite evidence to the contrary and out of keeping with the individual's social, religious, educational and cultural background.

Delusional perception: A new delusion that forms in response to a real perception without any logical sense. It is one of Schneider's first rank symptoms of schizophrenia.

Dementia: A syndrome of generalized decline of memory, intellect and personality, without impairment of consciousness, leading to functional impairment.

Dependence syndrome: Prolonged, compulsive substance use leading to addiction, tolerance and the potential for withdrawal syndromes.

Depersonalization: Feeling of detachment from the normal sense of self.

Depot: Long-acting, slow release medications given intramuscularly to improve adherence (e.g. certain antipsychotics).

Depression: A mood disorder characterized by a persistent low mood, loss of pleasure and/or lack of energy.

Derealization: The feeling that surroundings or people are experienced as unreal.

Disinhibition: A lack of restraint manifested in disregard for social conventions, impulsivity, and poor judgement.

Dissociation: A process of 'separating off' certain memories from normal consciousness (feature of dissociative disorder).

Diurnal mood variation: The patient's low mood is more pronounced during certain times of the day (usually in the morning).

Dizygotic twins: Twins formed after fertilization of two separate eggs.

Dopamine hypothesis: States that schizophrenia is secondary to over-activity of the mesolimbic dopamine pathways in the brain.

DSM: Published by the American Psychiatric Association and used in the USA for the diagnosis and classification of mental disorders. It is the American equivalent of ICD-10.

Dysarthria: A disorder in articulating speech.

Dysmorphophobia: Excessive preoccupation with barely noticeable or imagined defects in their physical appearance.

Dysphasia: Disorder in language (e.g. problems finding words).

Dysthymia: Depressive state for at least 2 years, which does not meet the criteria for a mild, moderate or severe depressive disorder.

Dystonia: Acute painful contractions (spasms) of muscles. May be a side effect of antipsychotic use.

Echolalia: Repetition of words. May be a feature of autism.

Elated mood: Elevation of mood.

Electroencephalogram (EEG): A measure of the electrical activity of the brain – gives information about the state of the patient's brain and their level of consciousness.

Encopresis: Deposition of normal faeces in inappropriate places in children who should have developed normal bowel control.

Enuresis: Involuntary voiding of urine in children who should have established bladder control. Can be linked to psychosocial stressors and organic causes must be excluded.

Erotomania: See *De Clérambault's syndrome*.

Euphoria: An exaggerated feeling of wellbeing – commonly associated with substance misuse.

Euthymic: An objective description of normal mood.

Executive function: Higher functions include planning, organization, problem solving, abstract thinking and decision making which may be lost in dementia.

Exposure and response prevention: A technique in which a patient is repeatedly exposed to a situation which causes them anxiety and they are prevented from performing the actions which lessen that anxiety – commonly used in OCD.

Extrapyramidal side effects: Potential problem with taking antipsychotics. Includes parkinsonism, akathisia, dystonia and tardive dyskinesia.

Flight of ideas: Speech difficult to understand as it switches rapidly from one loosely connected idea to another.

Folie à deux: A syndrome in which a delusional belief is transmitted from one individual to another such that they share the delusion.

Formal thought disorder: Abnormality of the way that thoughts are linked together.

Free association: Articulation of all thoughts that come to the mind. This is used in psychodynamic therapy.

Fregoli's syndrome: Delusion that strangers the individual meets are persecutors in disguise.

Graduated exposure: A technique in the treatment of phobias where one is exposed to a feared stimulus in a controlled manner with the end purpose of eradicating the fear.

Grandiosity: Inflated ideas about oneself. A feature of mania.

Hallucination: A false perception in the absence of an external stimulus.

Hyperarousal: An exaggerated response to normal stimuli (e.g. sound); a feature of PTSD.

Hypochondriasis: Misinterpretation of normal bodily sensations, leading to a non-delusional preoccupation of having a serious physical disease.

ICD-10: International classification of diseases is the standard diagnostic tool for clinical purposes, published by the World Health Organization.

Illusion: A false mental image produced by the misinterpretation of an external stimulus.

Insight: The extent to which the patient understands the nature of their condition.

Jamais vu: A failure to recognize events that have been encountered before.

Kleptomania: Inability to refrain from stealing, a differential diagnosis for OCD.

Knight's move thinking: A form of loosening of association where there is discourse consisting of a sequence of unrelated ideas.

Korsakoff's psychosis: Profound short-term memory loss characterized by confabulation, disorientation to time and personality change.

Labile mood: Refers to a fluctuating mood state.

Libido: Refers to sexual drive. May be reduced in depression.

Loosening of associations: A type of formal thought disorder involving the loss of the normal structure of thinking.

Malingering: Patient seeks advantageous consequences of being diagnosed with a medical condition. For instance, evading criminal prosecution or receiving benefits.

Mental capacity: The ability to take in information, process it in a structured way, weigh up the options, arrive at a decision and then communicate one's thoughts coherently.

Monoamine hypothesis: A deficiency in monoamine neurotransmitters causes depression.

Monozygotic twins: Two individuals with the same genetic makeup after a single egg was fertilized and split early in embryonic development.

Mood: Refers to a patient's sustained, subjective, experienced emotion over a period of time.

Multidisciplinary team (MDT): A group of professionals working together to ensure optimal patient management for their condition, with the patient at the centre of their treatment.

Munchausen's syndrome (factitious disorder): The individual wishes to adopt the 'sick role' in order to receive the care of a patient, for internal emotional gain.

Negative symptoms: Are deficits in association with schizophrenia and include apathy, blunting of affect, poverty of thought and speech, social isolation and poor self-care.

Neologism: Words or phrases devised by the patient which have no ordinary meaning.

Neuroleptic malignant syndrome: Rare but life-threatening condition seen in patients taking antipsychotic medications, characterized by pyrexia, muscle rigidity and autonomic instability.

Neurosis: Collective term for psychiatric disorders characterized by distress, that are non-organic, have a discrete onset and where delusions and hallucinations are absent.

Night terrors: Episode where individual (commonly a child) awakes suddenly from sleep, screaming in extreme distress and unresponsive to the efforts of others to console them.

Obsession: Unwanted, persistent, intrusive thoughts, images or urges that repeatedly enter the individual's mind in a stereotyped form.

Operant conditioning: States that consequences of actions (positive or negative) will affect future behaviour.

Othello syndrome: Delusion that their partner is being unfaithful without having any proof.

Overvalued idea (preoccupation): An isolated, preoccupying, strongly held belief derived through normal mental processes, which dominates a person's life and affects their actions.

Paraphrenia: Late onset schizophrenia. Positive symptoms occur in the absence of negative symptoms.

Passivity phenomenon: Belief that thoughts, sensations and actions being controlled by an external force.

Perseveration: Uncontrollable and often inappropriate repetition of a particular response (e.g. word or phrase).

Pervasive developmental disorder: A group of disorders characterized by delays in the development of socialization and communication skills (e.g. autism).

Phobia: An intense, irrational fear of an object, situation, place or person that is recognized as excessive (out of proportion to the threat) or unreasonable.

Positive symptoms: In relation to schizophrenia are active symptoms such as delusions, hallucinations and formal thought disorder.

Postnatal depression: Onset of depression after having a baby. Usually develops within 3 months of delivery and at its most extreme, patient can have intrusive thoughts of harming the baby.

Poverty of speech: Reduced speech. May be a feature of depression or dementia.

Premorbid personality: Personality or character prior to the onset of psychiatric illness.

Pressure of speech: Speech is abnormally fast as if there are too many ideas to verbalize at a given moment in time. May be a feature of mania.

Prion disease: A prion is a particle that does not contain DNA or RNA. Known to cause fatal diseases of the brain with spongiform degeneration. CJD is an example.

Prodrome: A symptom or group of symptoms indicating the onset of a disease.

Pseudodementia: Poor concentration and impaired memory are common in depression in the elderly population.

Pseudohallucination: As with hallucination but recognized by the individual as unreal.

Psychomotor agitation: Excessive activity or restlessness.

Psychomotor retardation: Slowing of movements or speech.

Psychosis: A mental state in which reality is greatly distorted.

Puerperal psychosis: Development of psychotic symptoms in the post-partum period (usually occurs within 3 weeks).

Purging: Compensatory weight loss behaviours in bulimia nervosa, e.g. self-induced vomiting.

Rapid cycling: A category of bipolar disorder with a poor prognosis.

Risk assessment: In a psychiatric context it is assessing the risk of self-harm, suicide and/or risk to others.

Rumination: Repetitively mulling over the same thoughts to the extent that other mental activity is impaired. A feature of PTSD.

Russell's sign: Calluses on the back of the hand indicative of self-induced vomiting and therefore a feature of bulimia nervosa.

Schizoaffective disorder: Characterized by both symptoms of schizophrenia and a mood disorder (depression or mania) in the same episode of illness.

Schizophrenia: Characterized by hallucinations, delusions and thought disorders which lead to functional impairment.

Schneider's first rank symptoms: If present, are strongly suggestive of schizophrenia (delusional perception, third person auditory hallucinations, thought interference, passivity phenomenon).

Selective mutism: Marked selectivity in speaking depending upon the social situation.

Serotonin syndrome: A rare but life-threatening complication of increased serotonin activity (e.g. with SSRI use).

Sick role: Refers to sickness and the rights and obligations of those affected. In somatoform disorders this role may be adopted for personal gain.

Social learning theory: Behaviour is learnt based on observation and imitation.

Somatic symptoms: Symptoms relating to the physical body (e.g. palpitations, dyspnoea).

Stress-vulnerability model: Predicts that schizophrenia occurs due to environmental factors interacting with a genetic predisposition.

Suicidal ideation: Recurrent thoughts about taking one's own life.

Suicide: A fatal act of self-harm initiated with the intention of ending one's own life.

Sundowning: In delirium, cognition often fluctuates and is more impaired at night compared to in the day, a feature referred to as sundowning.

Tangentiality: Diversion from original train of thought but no return to it.

Tardive dyskinesia: Late onset choreoathetoid movements (abnormal, involuntary movements) may be a result of antipsychotic use.

Testamentary capacity: Ability or competency of a person to make a will. May be impaired in dementia and psychiatrists of the elderly may be asked to assess this.

Thought blocking: Sudden cessation to flow of thoughts.

Thought broadcast: The belief that thoughts are audible to others or being broadcast (e.g. on television, radio) to the public.

Thought insertion: Belief that thoughts are being put into the mind from an outside agency.

Thought withdrawal: Belief that thoughts are being extracted from the mind by external agency.

Tics: Repeated, sudden, involuntary, irregular movements involving a group of muscles.

Tolerance: Need for increasing quantity of substance to produce desired effects.

Transference: In the context of psychodynamic psychotherapy, refers to the patient's relationship with the therapist in connection to previous relationships held with others.

Wernicke's encephalopathy: An acute encephalopathy which may be seen in chronic alcoholism, due to thiamine deficiency, presenting with delirium, nystagmus, ophthalmoplegia and ataxia.

Withdrawal syndrome: Physical or psychological effects from cessation of a substance after prolonged, repeated or high use.

Word salad: Speech that is reduced to senseless repetition of sounds or phrases.

Yerkes–Dodson law: States that anxiety can be beneficial up to a plateau of optimal functioning.

Appendix A

Answers to exam-style questions

1. **Answer: B**

   The three individuals are talking about him in the third person and therefore he is experiencing third person auditory hallucinations. The patient has also heard the radio presenter talking directly to him, and this would be a second person auditory hallucination not a delusion of reference. In delusions of reference the patient would hear what anyone hears when listening to the radio, but derive a delusional meaning from this. In persecutory delusions, patients believe that other people are conspiring against them in order to inflict harm or destroy their reputation and this is certainly not present. Pseudo-hallucinations would be recognized by the individual as unreal but there is no evidence to suggest this.

2. **Answer: C**

   Although the trigger may be the death of her mother and some could argue that this is an adjustment disorder, she meets the criteria for a depressive illness. She has two core symptoms, low mood and anhedonia, and has two other symptoms described, early morning wakening and loss of appetite. This therefore meets the criteria for mild depression (see *ICD-10: Classification of depression*). ICD-10 does not classify bereavement reactions. However, following bereavement, or any life event, if the individual meets the criteria for a depressive disorder, this diagnosis and treatment should be followed. If the bereavement is an important factor, bereavement counselling may be an appropriate psychological intervention.

   > **ICD-10 Classification of depression**
   >
   > **Mild depression:** 2 core symptoms + 2 other symptoms.
   > **Moderate depression:** 2 core symptoms + 3–4 other symptoms.
   > **Severe depression:** 3 core symptoms + ≥4 other symptoms.
   > **Severe depression with psychosis:** 3 core symptoms + ≥4 other symptoms + psychosis.

3. **Answer: D**

   It is not possible to say he has bipolar affective disorder, as we don't know if he has had a previous episode of mania or depression. His beliefs about his blood are probably grandiose delusions and therefore he would be classed as suffering from mania with psychosis (see *Fig. 3.3.2*).

4. **Answer: A**

   He has only had the symptoms for 2 weeks so cannot yet be diagnosed with paranoid schizophrenia, despite having first rank symptoms (remember symptoms have to be present for at least 1 month). For schizoaffective disorder you need to meet the criteria for schizophrenia and an affective disorder in the same episode. He is not suffering from a delusional disorder as in this disorder, patients present with delusions but no accompanying prominent hallucinations, but he has third person auditory hallucinations. No information has been given about mood symptoms to diagnose a severe depressive disorder.

5. **Answer: D**
    He is describing a thought being placed into his head that belongs to someone else (thought insertion). With thought withdrawal, patients believe their own thoughts are being taken away from them by someone else and in thought broadcast, patients believe that their thoughts are being heard out loud. He is clearly becoming paranoid about this being a trap, and he may have a secondary persecutory delusion.

6. **Answer: D**
    This is a classic description of social phobia, or fear of scrutiny by other people. To rule out agoraphobia you would want to know whether she struggles to go out. In social phobia individuals are able to function in crowds, but struggle in more intimate social situations, or when public speaking. Vomiting phobia or emetophobia is an intense, irrational fear of vomiting including fear of vomiting in a public place, fear of seeing vomit or fear of seeing the action of vomiting. Generalized anxiety disorder is a chronic disorder in which the patient is in a constant state of high anxiety; conversely in this patient, her anxiety is attributable only to social events.

7. **Answer: A**
    The description above is for panic disorder, which is causing significant problems for the individual, and is beginning to lead to avoidance. Benzodiazepines should probably be avoided and are not going to treat the underlying condition. Antidepressants such as SSRIs or TCAs could be used, depending on patient choice but are not given in the options. CBT is the most appropriate treatment from the list. CBT should be offered in primary care and a referral to see a psychiatrist is unwarranted at the present time. Further investigation to rule out an organic cause of anxiety (e.g. hyperthyroidism) is warranted, but further ECGs when this has been done in the Emergency Department are unlikely to reveal any new abnormalities.

8. **Answer: B**
    The symptoms of OCD need to be present for 2 weeks, not 1. While it is important to check about a co-morbid history of depression, a family history and his insight, these will not help to confirm the diagnosis of OCD. However, the diagnostic guidelines for OCD do include checking that the patient recognizes the thoughts as his own. Individuals with OCD are often very frustrated that they know the thoughts are their own, know the thoughts are irrational, but struggle to resist these thoughts because of the unpleasant physical anxiety symptoms this causes.

9. **Answer: D**
    All of the symptoms listed are possible in PTSD. Patients will often have co-morbid depression with low mood, anhedonia, etc. However, flashbacks, which include repeated reliving of the accident, are common, as is a state of autonomic hyperarousal with an exaggerated startle reaction. He may be on edge walking on the pavement and you may see him being easily startled at road noises. Nightmares are also common, which can affect sleep.

10. **Answer: B**
    There is no past history and the description is of a woman with a severe depression, with a possible depressive psychosis. First-line treatment would be with an SSRI and not with tricyclic antidepressants. Given the patient is struggling to concentrate during a brief assessment with her GP, she will not currently be suitable for CBT. An antipsychotic may be appropriate, although we would need more information; however, this again is not first-line. In this situation, watching and waiting would not be appropriate as she is at risk of remaining severely depressed or even becoming suicidal if not treated. This patient may need referral to secondary care, perhaps to home treatment, but that is not an option given.

11. **Answer: B**

    This man has bipolar affective disorder as he has had previous episodes of mania. It would therefore be best to avoid any of the antidepressants. Lamotrigine can be used as a mood stabilizer for bipolar depression and is therefore the most appropriate option from the list. CBT may be an appropriate longer-term treatment, but again not in combination with an antidepressant. Antidepressants are less effective in bipolar disorder than in unipolar depression and they can also trigger manic or hypomanic episodes. With active suicidal thoughts you may wish to limit prescriptions to 1 week to limit access to medication.

12. **Answer: A**

    This is a challenging question. Discharge home may be appropriate with more information, but only with urgent (same-day) home treatment. However, this is potentially a high risk situation, and the options C, D and E do not offer the level of support needed. All of the follow-up options will not be immediate and will take several weeks, during which the patient and his wife will be left alone. That leaves the admission options. It can be argued that he is 'passively accepting' treatment and therefore may lack capacity to consent to admission and treatment, and a Mental Health Act assessment may be the most appropriate course of action, even if after this the decision is to admit the patient informally to hospital.

13. **Answer: D**

    BMI = weight (kg) ÷ [height (m)]²
    BMI = 42 ÷ [1.6 × 1.6]
    BMI = 16.4
    Within the ICD-10 classification for anorexia nervosa, BMI would be expected to be 17.5 or less.

14. **Answer: C**

    To be clear that this is bulimia you must work out that the BMI is above 20, and therefore anorexia is unlikely. Although anorexics may sometimes binge and purge, the normal BMI goes strongly against this. Remember that over 50% of individuals with an eating disorder do not meet the ICD-10 criteria for AN and BN and are thus diagnosed with EDNOS. Also consider the physical consequences of repeated vomiting which can include biochemical and metabolic, as well as structural problems and oesophageal tears. The cause of this woman's presentation is probably a Mallory–Weiss tear due to repeated vomiting.

15. **Answer: B**

    In dissociative fugue there is a loss of memory (like in dissociative amnesia), but there is also an apparently purposeful journey away from home, or the place of work, during which self-care is maintained. Although there is no memory for the journey afterwards, during the journey the individual may present normally to others. In dissociative stupor there is profound reduction in, or absence of voluntary movements, speech and normal responses to stimuli. This is not a case of malingering as there is no evidence that this person is seeking advantageous consequences of being diagnosed with a medical condition. Similarly, there is no evidence that the patient is adopting a sick role for internal emotional gain (factitious disorder).

16. **Answer: E**

    In this situation the patient is presenting with symptoms with no physical cause, which is probably a somatization disorder. In hypochondriacal disorder the patient would present with a concern about a specific illness, e.g. Crohn's disease. There is no evidence of secondary gain which would point towards a diagnosis of malingering, and there is no evidence that the individual is consciously producing these symptoms, which would point towards factitious disorder.

17. Answer: B
Wernicke's encephalopathy is caused by a severe thiamine deficiency (vitamin B_1), and presents with a classical set of symptoms: delirium, nystagmus, ophthalmoplegia and ataxia. It requires urgent treatment with parenteral thiamine to prevent progression to Korsakoff's psychosis. Korsakoff's psychosis is a profound (often irreversible) short-term memory loss characterized by confabulation (the unconscious filling of gaps in memory with imaginary events) and disorientation to time.

18. Answer: B
With the amount of alcohol being consumed, the patient will require a high dose of benzodiazepines (often chlordiazepoxide), gradually reducing over 5–7 days, depending on the local protocol. The patient may be vitamin B deficient, and to prevent Wernicke's encephalopathy, Pabrinex injections should be considered, as oral thiamine and Vitamin B tablets may not be sufficient. These oral supplements should be considered long term after Pabrinex injections.

19. Answer: B
Remember that the six features of dependence syndrome can be recalled using the mnemonic Drug Problems Will Continue To Harm: Desire/compulsion to consume substance, Preoccupation with substance (neglect of alternative pleasures), Withdrawal effects, Control impaired, Tolerance increased, Harmful effects known but continues to persist. A diagnosis of dependence syndrome can be made if at least three of these six factors are present together.

20. Answer: D
This is a classic description of an individual with a schizoid personality, who has no interest in friends or normal social contacts, including relationships. Without any history of positive symptoms of psychosis such as hallucinations, delusions and thought disorder it would be difficult to say this is a case of paranoid schizophrenia. Individuals with a paranoid personality are suspicious, bear grudges, and usually have relationships, although these are often difficult to maintain because of the suspiciousness. There is no evidence at present to suspect an autistic spectrum disorder, and no evidence of a social phobia. Indeed, individuals with social phobia may struggle with relationships but find this frustrating and distressing.

21. Answer: C
A clear dissocial picture, with an individual who appears to accept no responsibility for his behaviour and actions, with problems dating back to adolescence. In the DSM classification, this would be an antisocial personality disorder, but in ICD-10 the term used is dissocial. Individuals with a paranoid personality are suspicious, bear grudges, and usually have relationships, although these are often difficult to maintain because of the suspiciousness. Self-harm is more common in emotionally unstable personality disorder (borderline subtype), but the rest of the history is more convincing for dissocial difficulties.

22. Answer: D
In this situation there is no immediate severe risk. Self-harm will continue in the short and medium term as it is being used as a coping strategy. The most appropriate treatment is most likely the group psychotherapy. An admission to a psychiatric hospital is unlikely to improve the current situation, and may make the situation worse. Given that she is already seeing a psychiatrist and has an appointment in 5 days, it is most appropriate to contact them, and the psychotherapist. Decisions about other support should be left to the existing care team in discussion with the patient, and not be made in a crisis situation. It may be appropriate to refer her to the Home Treatment/Crisis Team, but that option is not available. It would be inappropriate to prescribe from the Emergency Department, and there may be a risk that this prescription could then be used to self-harm. Although it may be tempting to ask people to stop self-harming, this is a gross over-simplification of the behaviour, and is unlikely to effect any change.

23. **Answer: C**

    C is the best answer in the first instance. This is probably an acute confusional state (delirium) on a background of early dementia. This could be caused by the infection, hypoxia, or another cause. Ensure his oxygen saturations are adequate, and move him to a well-lit side room. Ensure that when nurses are in his room they only talk to him, and they speak in a calm and clear manner. Benzodiazepines would not be appropriate, as these may lower his oxygen saturations by causing respiratory depression. Haloperidol may be appropriate, but it would not be the first action you take to manage the situation and may be used at very low dose if the environmental and nursing measures do not safely manage his agitation and he poses a risk to himself or others. Furthermore, 10 mg of haloperidol is a very large dose, and should not be used, especially in an individual who has not had antipsychotics before, and never in a patient of this age, in this situation. A dose of 0.5 mg haloperidol may be more appropriate.

24. **Answer: B**

    The picture of disorientation to time and short-term memory loss would suggest Alzheimer's. There are no features to suggest a frontal lobe dementia, such as worsening of social behaviour, disinhibition (reduced control over one's behaviour), apathy/restlessness, repetitive behaviour or changes in personality. Furthermore, memory is usually preserved in frontal lobe dementia in its early stages. The incident at night may be an illusion, and is not necessarily suggestive of a Lewy body dementia, which typically presents with visual hallucinations. One bottle of wine each week, spread across the week is within the safe limits of drinking set by the UK government, and therefore this is less likely to be alcoholic dementia, although you would still advise her to reduce this. The only vascular risk factor is hypertension, but the clinical picture is more suggestive of Alzheimer's.

25. **Answer: E**

    $$\text{Alcohol units} = \frac{\text{strength (\% alcohol by volume)} \times \text{volume (ml)}}{1000}$$

    $$\text{Alcohol units} = \frac{[40 \times 700] + [10 \times 5000]}{1000}$$

    Alcohol units = 78 units each day.

26. **Answer: B**

    Mild intellectual disability: IQ 50–69
    Moderate intellectual disability: IQ 35–49
    Severe intellectual disability: IQ 20–34
    Profound intellectual disability: IQ difficult to measure but less than 20
    Pervasive developmental disorder: a descriptive term for conditions including autism.

27. **Answer: A**

    The best answer is A. He is presenting with inflexibility, communication problems, and a seeming lack of being able to understand other people, all of which may point to an autism spectrum disorder. It is best to avoid the diagnosis of a personality disorder in a 17-year-old, and we would need to know more before starting to think about a schizoid or dissocial personality. There is no evidence of psychosis such as hallucinations and delusions, but social withdrawal may represent a prodromal phase.

28. **Answer: B**

    B is the best answer from the list. An ECG is important as antipsychotics do have cardiac side effects including prolonged QTc interval which can predispose to torsades de pointes. Atypical antipsychotics cause metabolic syndrome and can lead to significant weight gain and therefore measurement of BMI, waist circumference and blood glucose and lipids at baseline, and then at regular intervals, is important.

29. Answer: E

Lithium is nephrotoxic and excreted via the kidneys and so U&Es are measured at baseline and every 6 months. It is not metabolized by the liver, therefore liver function tests are not needed. Lithium levels are important as lithium works within a narrow therapeutic window (normal limit = 0.4–1 mmol/L), and if levels are high (>1.5 mmol/L) it is extremely toxic, and can cause seizures, coma and even death. Lithium also damages the thyroid and therefore TFTs need to be monitored at baseline and every year.

30. Answer: E

The only absolute contraindication is E. The other four are relative contraindications, and a decision would have to be made about the risk of progressing with ECT versus the benefits of treatment. With options A–D early discussion with the anaesthetist, and appropriate further investigations and interventions may be considered.

31. Answer: E

Based on the symptoms described above, clozapine is the next appropriate step. Clozapine is licensed as a third-line treatment for schizophrenia and it is the only antipsychotic that has evidence that it is more effective than other antipsychotics. It should only be prescribed after failing to respond to two other antipsychotics (treatment-resistant schizophrenia). There may be reasons why clozapine is not prescribed, which might include poor compliance with oral medication; however, it should be considered. If it is not appropriate an alternative antipsychotic will be needed. The choice of oral versus depot will depend on compliance issues. Given that the patient has not wanted to consider CBT, unless he can be persuaded to agree to this he cannot be forced into having talking therapies, and in this situation, it is unlikely to be effective.

32. Answer: A

The patient is describing four symptoms of the dependence syndrome: a desire to take the substance, difficulties in controlling the substance-taking behaviour (buying from the internet), withdrawal symptoms (sweats, shakes and physically unwell) and tolerance (needing bigger doses to get the same effect). Certain drugs can cause a dependence syndrome, e.g. alcohol, opiates and benzodiazepines. Lorazepam is a benzodiazepine and can rapidly cause a dependence syndrome.

33. Answer: B

Please note the location is Birmingham so the Mental Health Act 1983, as applied in England and Wales would be used. There is separate legislation for Scotland and Northern Ireland. You cannot use a section 5(4) or section 5(2) of the Mental Health Act 1983 in an Emergency Department. A patient needs to be admitted to hospital for these powers to be used. This rules out answers A, D and E. B is the best answer given that he appears to pose an immediate risk to himself as a result of his mental state and therefore it would be best to try to prevent him from leaving. If he does leave, C would still not be appropriate. Whilst you would want his parents to keep him under observation in this situation you would also contact the police to find him. The police could use section 136 of the Mental Health Act if they feel he is acting in a mentally disordered way in a public place, and take him to a place of safety for assessment.

34. Answer: D

When assessing capacity the first question you should ask yourself is 'Does the person have an impairment of the mind or brain, or a disturbance of mental function?' A severe phobia in this situation is an impairment of the mind that could impact on her ability to weigh up a decision. In this situation it can be argued that the patient lacks capacity. If a decision is taken that she lacks capacity, her husband can be consulted, but he cannot make decisions for her unless he has a medical lasting power of attorney (power of attorney can be over medical matters or finances), which the scenario does not describe. B is not correct, as the unborn baby has no legal status until outside the womb.

35. Answer: D

The description above is of a patient with a severe depressive disorder. She has ideas, possibly delusions of guilt relating to her husband's death. These depressive cognitions may impact on her ability to weigh up a decision. Therefore, it can be argued that she lacks capacity, and in her best interests the overdose can be treated. Remember that the Mental Health Act can only be used to treat psychiatric but not medical illness and therefore the Mental Capacity Act has to be utilized. She will, however, need psychiatric follow-up, which might include an admission and treatment for her mental health condition, possibly under the Mental Health Act.

36. Answer: C

The description may fit with a patient who has become depressed, is tearful, not engaging in activities, neglecting herself, has lost weight, and is struggling to sleep. Indeed, patients with Alzheimer's disease can also have non-cognitive symptoms of depression. A trial of an antidepressant would therefore be most appropriate. Options A, B and E will lead to sedation only and will not treat the underlying cause of depression. Changing her anti-dementia medication to a stronger medication such as memantine may help with memory but is unlikely to have an effect on her depressive symptoms.

37. Answer: C

The 'omnimicrotask' may be an example of a neologism. These can be new words created by the patient, or an everyday word used in an unusual way by the patient. The repetition of words or phrases is an example of perseveration. Circumstantiality is where thinking and speech are filled with unnecessary trivial details. Knight's move thinking is a form of formal thought disorder where there do not appear to be links between ideas in speech. Dysarthria is a problem with the articulation of speech seen in many different disorders, e.g. stroke.

38. Answer: C

This is a classical description of fragile X syndrome. It will be important as you approach finals to review all of your basic sciences, including genetics, as these conditions are easy to test, both in SBA and clinical examinations. Klinefelter's is 47 XXY, but intelligence is usually normal. Prader–Willi usually presents in childhood, with the best known feature being chronic and excessive hunger, leading to obesity, although incomplete sexual development is usually seen rather than the macro-orchidism described. Asperger's is a form of autism, and does not present with the other features.

39. Answer: E

The tuberoinfundibular pathway, when blocked, can cause raised prolactin levels, which in turn has a number of effects. This includes abnormal lactation, changes to menstrual cycle including amenorrhoea, and sexual dysfunction. A–D are all dopaminergic pathways. Antipsychotics work on the mesolimbic and mesocortical dopamine pathways to inhibit positive and negative symptoms of schizophrenia, respectively. Antipsychotics cause EPSE via the nigrostriatal pathway. E is not a dopaminergic pathway as its name suggests. Again in finals, basic sciences including neuroanatomy can be tested and this needs to be reviewed.

40. Answer: B

This question tests your knowledge of the roles and responsibilities of the multidisciplinary team. The OT may be best placed to coordinate his care from the list given. He needs adaptations to support him with his ADL at home. The psychiatrist may only see him every 6 months to monitor his Alzheimer's disease (hippocampal atrophy), and the rheumatologist likewise for the arthritis. The GP would be next best placed to coordinate the community care options needed. The physiotherapist does not currently have a role from the scenario described.

Appendix B

Answers to self-assessment questions

3.2 Depressive disorder

1. Anhedonia (lack of enjoyment). *(1 mark)*

2. She has two core symptoms (low mood >2 weeks, anergia) and four other symptoms (reduced concentration, weight loss, feelings of worthlessness and hopelessness). This is indicative of moderate depression. *(1 mark)*

3. Any four of the following: diurnal variation in mood *(1 mark)*, early morning wakening *(1 mark)*, loss of libido *(1 mark)*, psychomotor retardation *(1 mark)*, weight loss *(1 mark)*, and loss of appetite *(1 mark)*.

4. In a woman of this age, it is very important to rule out thyroid dysfunction as it can present very similarly *(1 mark)*. It is therefore necessary to carry out thyroid function tests (TFTs) including TSH, free T_3 and T_4 *(1 mark)*.

5. First-line antidepressants are selective serotonin reuptake inhibitors (SSRIs) *(1 mark)*. An example can include any of the following *(1 mark)*: citalopram, escitalopram, fluoxetine, paroxetine, sertraline, fluvoxamine.

6. Treatment-resistant depression *(1 mark)*, suicidal ideation *(1 mark)*, life-threatening depression, e.g. when the patient refuses to eat or drink *(1 mark)*, psychomotor retardation or stupor *(1 mark)*.

3.3 Bipolar affective disorder

1. Bipolar or bipolar affective disorder *(1 mark)*.

2. Any six of the following *(1/2 mark for each, total = 3 marks)*: hypomania, mania, cyclothymia, schizoaffective disorder, an organic presentation including hyper-/hypothyroidism, Cushing's disease, cerebral tumour (e.g. frontal lobe lesion with disinhibition), stroke, illicit drug ingestion (e.g. amphetamines, cocaine), acute drug withdrawal, side effect of corticosteroid use, or a personality disorder (histrionic or emotionally unstable would be most likely).

3. Any three of the following *(1 mark for each, total = 3 marks)*: grandiosity/inflated self-esteem, decreased sleep, pressure of speech, flight of ideas, distractibility, psychomotor agitation, involvement in pleasurable activities without consequential thought, e.g. spending sprees.

4. Hypomania is mildly elevated mood present for four or more days. Mania is as with hypomania but to a greater extent *(1 mark)*. Symptoms are present for >1 week, with complete disruption of work and social activities. In mania, they may have grandiose ideas and excessive spending could lead to debts *(1 mark)*. There may be sexual disinhibition and reduced sleep may lead to exhaustion in mania *(1 mark)*. Insight may be preserved in hypomania *(1 mark)*.

5. Any three of the following: lithium *(1 mark)*, valproate *(1 mark)*, carbamazepine *(1 mark)* and lamotrigine *(1 mark)*. They are teratogenic and should therefore ideally be avoided in women of child bearing age or, if required, should be used with extreme caution and careful monitoring *(1 mark)*.

4.2 Schizophrenia

1. Schizophrenia *(1 mark)*. Any four of the following differential diagnoses *(1/2 mark for each)*: acute psychotic episode, schizophrenia-like psychotic disorder, schizoaffective disorder, delusional disorder, psychotic depression, mania with psychosis, drug-induced psychosis, personality disorders (e.g. schizoid). The only unknown is the length of time he has had the symptoms.

2. Delusional perception ('He states he saw lightning and is now convinced that the FBI is after him and that federal agents gather information about his whereabouts') *(1 mark)*, thought interference ('He believes that they are trying to control his thoughts and movement') *(1 mark)*, third person auditory hallucinations ('He also hears them outside his house talking about how they will murder him') *(1 mark)*.

3. Any four of the following *(1 mark for each, total = 4 marks)*: Avolition ($\downarrow$ motivation), asocial behaviour, anhedonia, alogia (poverty of speech), blunted affect, cognitive deficits.

4. Any four of the following *(1 mark for each, total = 4 marks)*: FBC , ESR , TFTs, glucose, serum calcium, U&Es and LFTs , cholesterol, vitamin B_{12} and folate, urine drug test, ECG, EEG or CT scan.

5. Any of the following atypical antipsychotics *(1 mark)*: olanzapine, risperidone, quetiapine, amisulpride, aripiprazole. **NOTE:** Clozapine should not be given at this stage and would therefore be an incorrect answer. Any of the four following side effects *(1 mark for each, total = 4 marks)*: extrapyramidal side effects (e.g. parkinsonism), blurred vision, urinary retention, dry mouth, constipation, sedation, weight gain, postural hypotension, tachycardia, ejaculatory failure or sexual dysfunction, reduced bone mineral density, menstrual disturbances, breast enlargement, galactorrhoea, impaired glucose tolerance, hypercholesterolaemia, neuroleptic malignant syndrome, prolonged QT interval.

6. Any four of the following psychosocial interventions *(1 mark for each, total = 4 marks)*: CBT, psychoeducation, art therapy (e.g. music, dancing, drama), social skills training, social support groups, peer groups, supported employment programmes.

5.2 Generalized anxiety disorder

1. 6 months *(1 mark)*.

2. Any three of the following *(1 mark for each, total = 3 marks)*: FBC (for infection/anaemia), TFTs (hyperthyroidism), glucose (hypoglycaemia), ECG (may show sinus tachycardia).

3. Any six of the following *(1/2 mark for each, total = 3 marks)*: difficulty breathing, feeling of choking, nausea, abdominal distress, loose motions, hot flushes or cold chills, numbness or tingling, headache, muscle tension, aches or pains, restlessness, sensation of lump in throat (globus hystericus), difficulty swallowing (dysphagia).

4. The first-line drug treatment of choice is an SSRI *(1 mark)*.

5. Any two of the following *(1 mark for each, total = 2 marks)*: psychoeducation, CBT, applied relaxation, self-help methods, social support.

5.3 Phobic anxiety disorders

1. Specific phobia to flying *(1 mark)*.

2. Any two from *Fig. 5.3.1* *(1 mark for each, total = 2 marks)*.

3. Social phobia and agoraphobia *(1 mark)*. Social phobia is a marked fear or avoidance of social situations, or fear of acting in a way that will be embarrassing or humiliating *(1 mark)*. Agoraphobia is a fear of public spaces or fear of entering a public space from which immediate escape would be difficult in the event of a panic attack *(1 mark)*. **NOTE:** social phobia may occur with or without agoraphobia.

4. Self-help methods, CBT, benzodiazepines (short term) *(1 mark for each, total = 3 marks)*.

5. Symptoms of GAD occur most of the time whereas features of phobic anxiety disorders occur in response to particular situations *(1 mark)*. Commonly, agitation is an associated behaviour of GAD whereas avoidance of the particular situation typically occurs in phobic anxiety disorders *(1 mark)*. Concerning cognition, there is constant worry about everyday life events in patients with GAD whereas patients with phobic anxiety disorders only worry about or fear a particular situation *(1 mark)*.

5.4 Panic disorder

1. A panic attack/panic disorder *(1 mark)*.

2. Any three of the following *(1 mark for each, total = 3 marks)*: phaeochromocytoma, hyperthyroidism, hypoglycaemia, carcinoid syndrome, arrhythmias.

3. Symptoms in GAD present persistently, symptoms in panic disorder occur episodically and symptoms in phobic anxiety disorders occur in response to certain situations *(1 mark)*. GAD is associated with agitation; panic disorder is associated with a feeling of wanting to escape; phobic anxiety disorders are associated with avoidance of the particular situation *(1 mark)*. GAD patients commonly suffer from depression. Patients with panic disorder often have depression, agoraphobia and suffer from substance misuse. Those with phobic anxiety often suffer from substance misuse *(1 mark)*.

4. SSRIs are first-line for panic disorder *(1 mark)*.

5.5 Post-traumatic stress disorder

1. Any six of the following *(1/2 mark for each, total = 3 marks)*: flashbacks, vivid memories, recurring dreams, distress when exposed to similar circumstances as stressor, avoiding reminders of trauma (e.g. associated people or locations), excessive rumination about the trauma, inability to recall aspects of the trauma, irritability or outbursts, difficulty with concentration, difficulty with sleep, hypervigilance, exaggerated startle response.

2. 6 months *(1 mark)*.

3. Any two of the following *(1 mark for each, total = 2 marks)*: adjustment disorder requires a non-catastrophic event, whereas PTSD involves an exceptionally traumatic event *(1 mark)*. The symptoms in adjustment disorder must occur within 1 month of the event whereas PTSD must occur within 6 months *(1 mark)*. The symptoms in adjustment disorder must be present for less than 6 months. In PTSD, these symptoms may last longer *(1 mark)*.

4. CBT *(1 mark)*, eye movement desensitization and reprocessing *(1 mark)*.

5. Any two of the following *(1 mark for each, total = 2 marks)*: Any SSRI (most commonly paroxetine), mirtazapine, duloxetine, venlafaxine.

5.6 Obsessive–compulsive disorder

1. Obsessive–compulsive disorder/OCD *(1 mark)*.

2. Hypochondriacal disorder *(1 mark)*, anankastic personality disorder *(1 mark)*, schizophrenia *(1 mark)*, depression *(1 mark)*, generalized anxiety disorder *(1 mark)*.

3. 'Are these thoughts that you are getting repetitive and distressing?' *(1 mark)*; 'Are you aware that these thoughts are coming from your own mind?' *(1 mark)*; 'Do you feel anxious if you do not wash your hands and feet?' *(1 mark)*

4. In schizophrenia, patients often believe that the thoughts and hallucinations that they develop are real, whereas patients with OCD are aware that their obsessions are coming from their own mind *(1 mark)*.

5. SSRIs are the drug of choice in OCD *(1 mark)*. NICE recommends any of the following *(any two, 1 mark for each = 2 marks)*: fluoxetine, fluvoxamine, paroxetine, sertraline or citalopram.

6. Cognitive behavioural therapy *(1 mark)*. Exposure and response prevention *(1 mark)*.

5.7 Medically unexplained symptoms

1. Somatoform disorder *(1/2 mark)*, dissociative (conversion) disorder *(1/2 mark)*, factitious disorder *(1/2 mark)*, malingering *(1/2 mark)*.

2. Somatization disorder *(1 mark)* since she has had multiple and recurrent physical symptoms not explained by a physical illness *(1 mark)*.

3. Hypochondriacal disorder *(1 mark)*, somatoform autonomic dysfunction *(1 mark)* and persistent somatoform pain disorder *(1 mark)*.

4. In both malingering and factitious disorder (also known as Munchausen's syndrome) physical or psychological symptoms are intentionally produced, i.e. faked *(1 mark)*. In malingering, the patient seeks advantageous consequences of being diagnosed with a medical condition, e.g. financial gain *(1 mark)*. In factitious disorder, the individual wishes to adopt the 'sick role' in order to receive the care of a patient, for internal emotional gain (i.e. primary gain) *(1 mark)*.

6.1 Anorexia nervosa

1. BMI = weight (kg)/[height (m)]^2 = 42/(1.6^2) *(1 mark)* = 16.4 *(1 mark)*.

2. Anorexia nervosa *(1 mark)*. Any two of the following: bulimia nervosa *(1/2 mark)*, EDNOS *(1/2 mark)*, depression *(1/2 mark)*, hyperthyroidism *(1/2 mark)*.

3. Any four of the following *(1 mark for each)*: Fear of weight gain, Endocrine disturbances (e.g. amenorrhoea), Emaciated (abnormally low weight >15% below expected weight or BMI <17.5 kg/m^2), Deliberate weight loss, Distorted body image.

4. Any four of the following *(1 mark for each, total = 4 marks)*: hypokalaemia, hypotension, hypothermia, anaemia, cardiac failure, hypoglycaemia, osteoporosis, acute renal failure.

5. A bio-psychosocial approach should be adopted. She should be assessed medically to see whether she has any complications of AN, and this should be treated accordingly, ideally as an inpatient *(1 mark)*. She should be educated about her condition and need for nutrition *(1 mark)* and be offered long-term psychotherapy *(1 mark for any of the following)*: CBT, interpersonal therapy or family therapy. Access to voluntary organizations and self-help groups should also be offered *(1 mark)*. If she refuses treatment, the need for the Mental Health Act should be considered *(1 mark)*.

6.2 Bulimia nervosa

1. Bulimia nervosa *(1 mark)*. Anorexia nervosa *(1 mark)* and any of the following: EDNOS *(1 mark)*, depression *(1 mark)*, OCD *(1 mark)*.

2. Compensatory weight gain prevention behaviour *(1 mark)*, strong cravings *(1 mark)*, fear of fatness *(1 mark)* and binge eating *(1 mark)*.

3. Hypokalaemia *(1 mark)*. Can be tested quickly via a venous blood gas (although this can be inaccurate by up to 1 mmol/L) *(1 mark)*. Accurate testing would require a set of U&Es. *(1 mark)*

4. Any two of the following: pitted teeth *(1 mark)*, Russell's sign *(1 mark)*, enlargement of salivary glands *(1 mark)*, oesophageal (Mallory–Weiss) tears *(1 mark)*.

5. The management of BN is based on the bio-psychosocial model. A trial of antidepressant should be offered and can ↓ frequency of binge eating/purging *(1 mark)*. CBT for bulimia nervosa should also be offered *(1 mark)*; interpersonal psychotherapy is an alternative *(1 mark)*. Simple measures can be employed, such as a food diary to monitor eating/purging patterns, techniques to avoid bingeing (eating in company, distractions), small, regular meals *(1 mark)*.

7.1 Substance misuse

1. An opiate *(1 mark)* such as heroin.

2. Class A *(1 mark)*.

3. Naloxone *(1 mark)* Intravenous *(1 mark)*.

4. Any four of the following *(1 mark for each, total = 4 marks)*: compulsive need to consume drug, preoccupation with substance use, withdrawal state when substance ingestion is reduced or stopped, impaired ability to control substance-taking behaviour, increased tolerance to substance, persisting despite clear evidence to harmful effects.

5. Motivational interviewing *(1 mark)*, CBT *(1 mark)*, contingency management *(1 mark)*.

7.2 Alcohol abuse

1. Any four of the following *(1 mark for each, total = 4 marks)*: subjective awareness of compulsion to drink, avoidance or relief of withdrawal symptoms by further drinking, withdrawal symptoms, drink-seeking behaviour predominates, reinstatement after abstinence, narrowing of drinking repertoire.

2. Any of the two medical complications *(1/2 mark each)*: hepatitis, cirrhosis, hepatocellular carcinoma, peptic ulcer, oesophageal varices, oesophageal carcinoma, pancreatitis, hypertension, cardiomyopathy, arrhythmias, anaemia, thrombocytopenia, seizures, peripheral neuropathy, cerebellar degeneration, Wernicke's encephalopathy, Korsakoff's psychosis, head injury (secondary to falls). Any two of the following psychiatric complications *(1/2 mark each)*: morbid jealousy, self-harm and suicide, mood disorder, anxiety disorders, alcohol dementia, alcoholic hallucinosis, delirium tremens. Any two of the following social complications *(1/2 mark each)*: domestic violence, drink driving, employment difficulties, financial problems, homelessness, accidents, relationship problems.

3. Delirium tremens is a complication of alcohol withdrawal which usually develops between 24 hours to one week after alcohol cessation *(1 mark)*. It is characterized by perceptual abnormalities (hallucinations and/or illusions) *(1 mark)*, cognitive impairment *(1 mark)*, paranoid delusions *(1 mark)*, autonomic arousal *(1 mark)* (e.g. tachycardia, fever and increased sweating) and marked tremor *(1 mark)*.

4. High dose benzodiazepines (commonly chlordiazepoxide) are given initially *(1 mark)*, and the dose is then tapered down over roughly a one-week period *(1 mark)*.

8 Personality disorders

1. Emotionally unstable/borderline personality disorder *(1 mark)*.

2. Any six of the following *(1/2 mark for each, total = 3 marks)*: paranoid personality disorder, schizoid personality disorder, dissocial personality disorder, histrionic personality disorder, anankastic personality disorder, anxious (avoidant) personality disorder.

3. Any three of the following *(1 mark for each, total = 3 marks)*: callous, blame others, disregard for safety, remorseless, deceitful, impulsive tendency to violence.

4. CBT *(1 mark)*, psychodynamic therapy *(1 mark)*, dialectical behavioural therapy (DBT) *(1 mark)*.

9.1 Deliberate self-harm

1. Any three of the following *(1 mark for each, total = 3 marks)*: divorced/single/living alone, severe life stressors, harmful drug/alcohol use, less than 35 (age), chronic physical health problems, domestic violence or childhood maltreatment, socioeconomic disadvantage, psychiatric illness (e.g. depression, psychosis).

2. Any three of the following *(1 mark for each, total = 3 marks)*: genuine wish to die, seeking unconsciousness or pain as a means of temporary relief and escape from problems, trying to influence another person to change their views or behaviour, to punish oneself, to seek attention.

3. ABCDE approach *(1 mark)*, give IV N-acetylcysteine if above treatment line *(1 mark)*.

4. Acute liver failure *(1 mark)*.

5. Any three of the following *(1 mark for each, total = 3 marks)*: Was it planned? What method did they use? Was a suicide note left? Was the patient intoxicated with drugs or alcohol? Was the patient

alone? Were there any efforts to avoid discovery (e.g. waited until house empty)? Did the patient seek help after the attempt or were they found and brought in by someone else? How does the patient feel about the episode now? (regret? do they wish that they had succeeded?) How did they feel when they were found?

9.2 Suicide and risk assessment

1. Male *(1 mark)*, stress *(1 mark)*, medical conditions *(1 mark)*, depression *(1 mark)*.

2. Any four of the following risk factors *(1/2 mark for each, total = 2 marks)*: history of DSH, previous attempted suicide, psychiatric illness, family history of suicide, childhood abuse, age (middle aged), unemployed, low socioeconomic status, certain occupations, access to lethal means, low social support, living alone, institutionalized, single, widowed, divorced, recent life crisis.

3. Responsibility for someone else *(1 mark)*.

4. If high risk there is a possibility for him to be hospitalized informally or via the MHA *(1 mark)*. He should first be assessed by the Crisis team to see if he could be safely managed in the community with intensive input *(1 mark)*. He will need to be started on an SSRI, and consider CBT, and other support that may be available to him as a carer *(1 mark)*.

5. Any two of the following *(1 mark for each, total = 2 marks)*: Public education and discussion *(1 mark)*, reducing access to means of suicide *(1 mark)*, easy, rapid access to psychiatric care or support groups *(1 mark)*, e.g. Samaritans (who provide emergency 24 hour support), decreasing societal stressors, e.g. unemployment *(1 mark)*.

10.1 Delirium

1.

	Delirium	Dementia	
Sleep-wake cycle	Disrupted	Usually normal	*(1 mark)*
Attention	Markedly reduced	Normal/reduced	*(1 mark)*
Arousal	Increased/decreased	Usually normal	*(1 mark)*
Autonomic features	Abnormal	Normal	*(1 mark)*
Duration	Hours to weeks	Months to years	*(1 mark)*
Delusions	Fleeting	Complex	*(1 mark)*
Course	Fluctuating	Stable/slowly progressive	*(1 mark)*
Consciousness level	Impaired	No impairment	*(1 mark)*
Hallucinations	Common (especially visual)	Less common	*(1 mark)*
Onset	Acute/subacute	Chronic	*(1 mark)*
Psychomotor activity	Usually abnormal	Usually normal	*(1 mark)*

2. Any six of the following *(1/2 mark for each, total = 3 marks)*: infection, hypoxia, electrolyte disturbances, hypoglycaemia, nutritional deficiencies, stroke, MI, drugs (e.g. opioids, benzodiazepines, anticholinergics), alcohol withdrawal, head trauma, epilepsy, constipation, urinary retention, bladder catheterization, hyperthyroidism, hypothyroidism, hyperglycaemia, severe pain, sensory deprivation (for example leaving the person without spectacles or hearing aids), relocation (such as moving people with impaired cognition to unfamiliar environments), sleep deprivation.

3. Any of the following *(1/2 mark for each, total = 5 marks)*: urinalysis, FBC, U&Es, LFTs, calcium, glucose, CRP, TFTs, haematinics, ECG, CXR, blood culture and urine culture.

4. The Abbreviated Mental Test *(1 mark)* and Confusion Assessment Method tools *(1 mark)*, Mini-Mental State Examination *(1 mark)*.

5. Treat the underlying cause – in this case it is most likely to be infection and/or anaesthesia-related *(1 mark)*. Reassure and orientate patient *(1 mark)*. The patient should be provided with the appropriate environment, e.g. a quiet well-lit side room if practical *(1 mark)*, consistency in care and staff *(1 mark)*, encourage presence of friend/family member, optimize sensory acuity, e.g. glasses *(1 mark)*, well-lit room *(1 mark)*, orientation aids (clock, calendar) *(1 mark)*. Low dose sedatives should be used as a last resort, and may make the situation worse *(1 mark)*. **NOTE:** The presence of friend/family member will not be practical in the middle of the night.

10.2 Dementia

1. Alzheimer's disease *(1 mark)*.
2. Microscopic: neurofibrillary tangles *(1 mark)* and β-amyloid plaque formation *(1 mark)*. Macroscopic: cortical atrophy (commonly hippocampal) *(1 mark)* with widened sulci *(1 mark)* and enlarged ventricles *(1 mark)*.
3. Any five of the following *(1 mark for each, total = 5 marks)*: FBC, CRP, U&Es, calcium, LFTs, glucose, lipids, vitamin B_{12} and folate, TFTs, VDRL.
4. Moderate *(1 mark)*.
5. Any six of the following *(1/2 mark for each, total = 3 marks)*: Normal pressure hydrocephalus, intracranial tumours, chronic subdural haematoma, vitamin B_{12} deficiency, folic acid deficiency, thiamine deficiency, pellagra (niacin deficiency), Cushing's syndrome, hypothyroidism.
6. Any four of the following *(1 mark for each, total = 4 marks)*: Social support, increasing assistance with day-to-day activities, information and education, carer support groups, community dementia teams, home nursing and personal care, community services such as meals-on-wheels, befriending services, day centres, respite care and care homes. For non-cognitive and behavioural challenges – aromatherapy, massage, therapeutic use of music or animal-assisted therapy may be considered.
7. Any two of the following *(1 mark for each, total = 2 marks)*: donepezil, galantamine and rivastigmine. **NOTE:** Memantine should only be given to those with moderate Alzheimer's disease who are intolerant of or have a contraindication to acetylcholinesterase inhibitors, or those with severe Alzheimer's disease and therefore this is NOT a correct answer.

11.1 Autism

1. Autism/autism spectrum disorder *(1 mark)*.
2. Have they reached all their other milestones accordingly, e.g. 'Can he walk?' *(1 mark)*; 'Is there any family history of autism?' *(1 mark)*; 'Does he have any other medical conditions, e.g. visual or hearing impairment?' *(1 mark)*; 'Have you noticed him making any abnormal movements such as flapping his hands or walking on tiptoes?' or 'Does your child insist on the same toys, activities or foods?' *(1 mark)*
3. Impairment in social interaction *(1 mark)*, impairment of communication *(1 mark)* and restricted, stereotyped interests and behaviours *(1 mark)*.
4. Any three of the following *(1 mark for each, total = 3 marks)*: visual impairment, hearing impairment, sensory issues, infections, epileptic seizures, hyperkinetic disorder, pica, sleep disorders, constipation, PKU, fragile X, tuberous sclerosis, congenital rubella, CMV, toxoplasmosis.
5. Any four of the following *(1/2 mark for each, total = 4 marks)*: CBT, family support, access to self-help groups such as the National Autistic Society group, special schooling, social-communication intervention (e.g. play-based strategies), modification of environmental factors which initiate or maintain challenging behaviour.

11.2 Hyperkinetic disorder

1. Hyperkinetic disorder or attention deficit hyperactivity disorder *(1 mark)*.
2. Inattention *(1 mark)*, hyperactivity *(1 mark)* and impulsivity *(1 mark)*.

3. Any three types of questions that cover the three core features of hyperkinetic disorder (see *History box* in *Section 11.2*).

4. In severe hyperkinetic disorder in school-aged children, drug treatment is first-line with methylphenidate (Ritalin) being the usual choice *(1 mark)*. Atomoxetine is second-line *(1 mark)*. If this fails, dexamfetamine is the alternative when methylphenidate has been ineffective *(1 mark)*.

11.3 Learning disability

1. Any three of the following *(1 mark for each, total = 3 marks)*: palpebral fissure (up slanting), round face, occipital + nasal flattening, Brushfield spots (pigmented spots on iris), brachycephaly, epicanthic folds, mouth open + protruding tongue, strabismus (squint), sandal gap deformity.

2. Any five from *Table 11.3.1* *(1 mark for each, total = 5 marks)*.

3. Mild: IQ = 50–70 *(1 mark)*; moderate: IQ = 35–49 *(1 mark)*; severe: IQ = 20–34 *(1 mark)*.

4. Any four of the following *(1 mark for each, total = 4 marks)*: psychiatrist, speech and language therapist, specialist nurses, psychologist, occupational therapist, educational support, social worker, and paediatrician.

Appendix C

Figure acknowledgements

Fig. 2.2.4
Reproduced from http://gpuzzles.com/optical-illusion/sleeping-baby-cloud/

Fig. 5.7.5
Reproduced from http://theprivatetherapyclinic.co.uk/understanding-body-dysmorphic-disorder-bdd/

Fig. 6.1.2
Reproduced from www.health.com/health/gallery/0,,20665980_5,00.html

Fig. 6.2.2(a)
Reproduced from *Journal of Clinical Pediatric Dentistry* (2011) **36(2):** 155–160, P.R. Kavitha, P. Vivek, A.M. Hegde, 'Eating Disorders and their Implications on Oral Health – Role of Dentists'.

Fig. 6.2.2(b)
Reproduced courtesy of Dr Alfredo Aguirre (School of Dental Medicine, University at Buffalo, The State University of New York).

Fig. 6.2.2(c)
Loss of enamel from the inside of the upper teeth as a result of bulimia.
Licensed under the Creative Commons Attribution-Share Alike 4.0 International licence.
Additional attribution: James Heilman, MD
Available at: https://commons.wikimedia.org/wiki/File:BulemiaEnamalLoss.JPG

Fig. 7.2.2(a)
Reproduced with permission from http://thehappyhospitalist.blogspot.co.uk

Fig. 7.2.2(b)
Reproduced with permission from http://blog.mmenterprises.co.uk

Fig. 7.2.2(c)
Reproduced from www.kingstonlaser.co.uk/index.php?page=acp

Fig. 7.2.2(d)
Reproduced from www.plasticsurgeryhub.com.au/plastic-surgery-before-and-after-photos/gynaecomastia-male-breast-reduction-photo-gallery/

Fig. 9.1.2
Self-injury in the form of cutting.
Licensed under the Creative Commons Attribution-Share Alike 3.0 Unported licence.
Additional attribution: Hendrike
Available at: https://commons.wikimedia.org/wiki/File:Schnittwunden.JPG

Fig. 10.2.1
Reproduced from http://coloradodementia.org/2011/12/28/the-plaques-and-tangles-of-alzheimers/

Fig. 10.2.5
Reproduced with kind permission of Dr Julio Acosta-Cabronero, German Center for Neurodegenerative Diseases (DZNE).

Appendix C Figure acknowledgements

Index

Bold indicates main entry

De Clérambault's syndrome, 20, 239
Da Costa's syndrome, 81, 239
deliberate self-harm (DSH), 93, 118, **120–3**, 126, 169, 239
delirium, 5, 11, 17, 24, 44, 106–9, **131–6**
delirium tremens, **107**, 132, 189, 239
delusion, 12, **19–22**, 31, 37, 44–50, 55, 100, 107–8, 116, 127, 131–3, 177
    bizarre, 20, 49
    grandiose, **20**, 37–8, 45, 49
    hypochondriacal, 20
    infestation, 20
    mood congruent, 20
    nihilistic, see Cotard's syndrome
    paranoid, 20, 65, 100, 107–8, 205
    persecutory, 12, **20**, 31, 37–9, 45, 47, 49–50, 132
    primary, 20–1
    reference, 20, 47, 49–50, 100
    secondary, 20
delusional disorder, 4–5, **44–5**, 177
    induced, 44–5
    persistent, 44–5
delusional memory, 21
delusional perception, **21–2**, 47, 239
dementia, 3, 5, 11, 17, 44, 76, 132–4, **137–47**, 239
    alcohol-related, 106
    fronto-temporal, 17, 137–8, **141–3**, 145
    Lewy body, 137–8, 141, 146
    mixed, 138, 141
    vascular, 137–8, **140–3**, 145
dependence syndrome, 15, 98
depersonalization, **22**, 55, 59, 68, 100, 239
depot injection, 6, 51–2, **182**, 239
depression, 11–13, 17–18, 27, **29–34**, 36–8, 60–1, 72, 89, 93, 122, 127–8, 140–1, 143, 164, 167–8, 170–6, 185, 193, 205, 239, 241
    atypical, 30–1, 33
    masked, 33
    postnatal, 33, 167, 205, 241
    postschizophrenic, 48
Deprivation of Liberty Safeguard (DoLS), 197
derailment of thought, 19, 21

derealization, **22**, 55, 59, 68, 239
dexamfetamine, 157
dialectical behavioural therapy (DBT), 118, **169**
diamorphine, 99
diazepam, 189
disinhibition, 17, 37–9, 99, 107–8, 141, 239
dissociative
    amnesia, 79
    anaesthesia and sensory loss, 79
    convulsions, 79
    disorder, 68, **78–9**, 83, 166, 238–9
    fugue, 79
    motor disorders, 79
    stupor, 79
disulfiram, 110–11
diurnal variation in mood, 30, 33, 239
donepezil, 146
dosulepin, 174–5
Down's syndrome, 138, **159–61**
doxepin, 174–5
Driver and Vehicle Licensing Agency (DVLA), 145
DSM-V, 4, 37, 239
dysarthria, 18, 41, 138, 190, 239
dysmorphophobia, 76, **80–1**, 83, 239
dysphasia, 18, 140, 145, 239
dyspraxia, 157
dysthymia, 27–8, **33**, 166, 170, 239
dystonia, 17, **179–80**, 239

early intervention in psychosis team, 7
early morning wakening, 30
eating disorder not otherwise specified (EDNOS), **89**, 95
eating disorders, 57, 76, **86–96**, 164, 168
echolalia, 150, 239
ecstasy, 100, 102
Edward and Gross criteria, 106
electroconvulsive therapy (ECT), 8, 33, 40, 51, **192–4**
electroencephalogram (EEG), 143, 192–3
emotional numbing, 71
epilepsy, 13, 44, 50, 76, 131, 159, 187
episodic anxiety, 56, 68